# Garlic
### The Natural Remedy

Jim-

Trust Rodney
and use this for
your Rehab program.

Art & Theresa

# Garlic
## The Natural Remedy

**Karen Evennett**

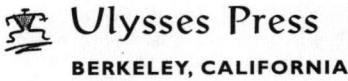
Ulysses Press
**BERKELEY, CALIFORNIA**

Copyright © 1998 Karen Evennett. All rights reserved under International and Pan-American Copyright Conventions, including the right to reproduce this book or portions thereof in any form whatsoever, except for use by a reviewer in connection with a review.

Published by: Ulysses Press
P.O. Box 3440
Berkeley, CA 94703-3440

Library of Congress Catalog Card Number: 97-61590

ISBN: 1-56975-097-1

First published as *Garlic: Natural Remedies* by Sheldon Press

Printed in Canada by Transcontinental Printing

10 9 8 7 6 5 4 3 2 1

Editor: Mark Woodworth
Cover Design: B&L Design
Book Design: Sarah Levin
Cover Photograph: Super Stock
Editorial and production staff: Lily Chou, Natasha Lay
Typesetter: David Wells
Indexer: Sayre Van Young

Distributed in the United States by Publishers Group West and in Canada by Raincoast Books

This book has been written and published strictly for informational purposes, and in no way should it be used as a substitute for consultation with your medical doctor or health care professional. All facts in this book came from medical files, clinical journals, scientific publications, personal interviews, published trade books, self-published materials by experts, magazine articles, and the personal-practice experiences of the authorities quoted or sources cited. You should not consider educational material herein to be the practice of medicine or to replace consultation with a physician or other medical practitioner. The author and publisher are providing you with information in this work so that you can have the knowledge and can choose, at your own risk, to act on that knowledge. The author and publisher also urge all readers to be aware of their health status and to consult health professionals before beginning any health program, including changes in dietary habits.

All names and identifying characteristics of real persons have been changed in the text to protect their confidentiality.

# Contents

| 1 | Garlic—Why Is It So Special | 1 |
| 2 | Garlic for Your Health | 9 |
| 3 | Garlic as a Remedy for Common Ailments | 29 |
| 4 | Good Health and Garlic | 51 |
| 5 | Garlic Recipes | 75 |

*Further Reading* — *138*

*Index* — *139*

*About the Author* — *143*

# 1

# Garlic—Why Is It So Special?

BACK IN THE LATE 1960S MY great-aunt arrived for one of her annual visits and produced, from her handbag, a jar of garlic capsules, or "pearles," which she said she was using every day to keep her in good health. She died a few years ago, just a couple of months away from her hundredth birthday. Who can say if the garlic had any effect on Aunt Nancy's longevity? She also swore by her daily swim in the English Channel, and the apple and banana she had without fail for her breakfast.

## Garlic Throughout the Ages

The idea that garlic is a natural anti-aging agent—studies have shown that it can rejuvenate the arteries by 15 years—is one of its biggest selling points, and although Aunt Nancy seemed to be ahead of the times in taking it as a supplement in the 1960s, garlic is in fact one of the most ancient remedies around.

The Egyptologist Sir William Petrie traced its use back to 3750 B.C., well before the Pharaohs arrived in Egypt. And Pliny, the ancient Greek physician, named no fewer than 61 ailments that could be treated with garlic.

Writing his *Complete Herbal* in 1653, Nicholas Culpeper claimed that garlic is something of a cure-all:

> ...a remedy for all diseases and hurts. It provokes urine, and women's courses, helps the biting of mad dogs and other venomous creatures, kills worms in children, cuts and voids tough phlegm, purges the head, helps the lethargy, it is a good preservative against and a remedy for any plague, sore or foul ulcers....

But, by the beginning of the nineteenth century, garlic had gone into serious decline in Great Britain, and its popularity wasn't helped by Mrs. Beeton, who, in her Victorian cookbook, wrote that she considered garlic unsuitable as a cooking ingredient and only worth using for a light wipe around the salad bowl. She famously proclaimed: "The smell of garlic is generally considered offensive."

At the beginning of the twentieth century, those who got to hear about the benefits of garlic did so from foreign sources. In the First World War, the Russians used crushed garlic as a dressing for wounds, to protect against gangrene; and in the

Second World War, garlic came to be called "Russian penicillin," a nickname it retains to this day.

It's only in the last 20 years or so, with the growth of interest in complementary or holistic medicines and alternative or natural therapies, that garlic has started enjoying a new revival. So much so that, in 1994, a Garlic Information Center was established in Great Britain—and continues to flourish—in East Sussex, to promote the use of garlic as a treatment for everything from the common cold to coronary heart disease, high blood pressure, and poor circulation. And many of the uses of garlic that were once considered to be no more than old wives' tales (oddly enough, there appear to have been no "old husbands' tales"!) are now proven beyond reasonable doubt.

- Raw garlic contains water, fat, sugars, pectin, cellulose, mucilage, total ash, acid soluble ash, peptides, and proteins.

- Its mineral content includes selenium, sodium, potassium, iron, cobalt, zinc, nitrogen, calcium, chromium, sulfur, magnesium, phosphorus, copper, and iodine.

- It has the following vitamins: A, $B_1$, $B_2$, and C. These make it a superb antioxidant.

- Its principal active agent is allicin, which produces the characteristic garlic odor. It's not an ingredient, but rather is produced when the sulfur compound alliin reacts with the enzyme alliinase. (*Allium* may be familiar to you as the genus name for bulbous herbs of the lily family, including garlics, onions, chives, leeks, and shallots.)

## The Many Benefits of Garlic

I will be looking, over the course of this book, at the ways in which garlic can help our health, and, more importantly, how we should use it.

The following claims, from the Garlic Information Center, will give you some idea of why garlic is enjoying such a revival and why it has even been hailed as the medical salvation of the Western world.

- Chewing raw garlic every day is said to build up your strength.

- Garlic can help keep cholesterol levels normal.

- Garlic is a potent antibacterial agent and can kill some of the most resistant and harmful bacteria known to science.

- Garlic is the only antibiotic that kills bacteria even while it encourages digestion.

- Garlic is an excellent antioxidant that can reduce harmful free radicals circulating in your body.

- Garlic may keep your blood cells healthy in the presence of various pollutants such as lead, mercury, copper, and aluminum.

- Taken regularly, garlic can help keep your circulation healthy.

- Studies confirm that garlic can keep blood pressure down.

- Garlic has been shown to increase blood flow to the nail-fold capillaries around the fingernails.

- Improved circulation to the arteries in the eye has also been demonstrated as a result of taking garlic.

- Studies have shown that garlic can kill deadly human parasites including *Entamoeba histolytica* and *Giardia lamblia*.

- Garlic is the richest source of organically bound selenium, which has been shown to provide some protection against heavy-metal poisoning.

- Garlic is a known carminative, stimulating the secretion of digestive juices and expelling gas from the alimentary canal so as to relieve colic.

- Many people have reported that regularly taking garlic in any form has kept them free of colds, over years.

- Garlic can kill the bacteria responsible for skin, lung, throat, and mouth infections.

- Researchers have shown that garlic can stimulate the number of natural "killer" cells in our bodies that help rid us of harmful invading organisms.

- It's said that as little as half a clove of garlic a day may be enough to keep cholesterol levels normal.

- Garlic may prevent stomach bugs of various sorts and help get rid of diarrhea.

- Taking a large dose of garlic as you feel a cold coming on can often stop it completely.

- Garlic is good for diabetics, as it will help normalize the level of body fats that can get out of control.

## Old Wives' Tales or Modern Medicine?

The following remedies are suggested by the Garlic Information Center:

- Take garlic tablets when you're at the lake or out on a hike through the woods, to help ward off mosquitos.

- Rub garlic paste over an aching tooth and it will remove the pain.

- Put a clove of garlic in a child's shoe to deter whooping cough (the smell will be excreted through the lungs).

- Use a swab of garlic to stop a nosebleed.

- Garlic can be used to calm bites and stings. Crush three cloves of garlic, mix with some warm water, and dab it on the affected parts.

- Mix garlic with lard and apply to your skin to help pimples and boils disappear.

- As a remedy for earache, soak a peeled clove of garlic in olive oil for a few minutes and place it in your ear, stopping it up with a cotton ball or two. The ache will vanish.

- For mouth ulcers (canker sores), chop the end off a clove of garlic, dip it into a container of natural yogurt, and apply it directly to the mouth ulcer. It will sting, but only for a moment.

- Gargle with crushed cloves of garlic mixed with brewed sage and warm water, to clear the throat.

- Try rubbing crushed garlic on your skin before sunbathing, as it's thought to be a good sun shield, but if you feel any burning from the sun (or the garlic), cover up immediately.

- Soak your fingernails in warm water containing a cut clove of garlic to keep them strong and prevent splitting.

- Scorpion bites produce harmful enzymes that can be treated by cutting up a clove of garlic and spreading it on the wound.

- Use fresh Chinese garlic for infections, digestive problems, and bronchitis, but use garlic tablets for circulation and to aid blood pressure and cholesterol levels.

- Raw garlic is often useful for treating acne and eczema, as it tends to remove the internal impurities that cause the problem.

- Use garlic as an inhalant for nasal congestion. Take three or four cloves, crush them, and add a little cider vinegar. Then pour on a pint of boiling water and inhale the fumes.

- Even when diluted by a ratio of 1 in 20, dried garlic powder can still kill the salmonella bug.

- If you have a warty skin lesion (known as a verruca), try cutting a thin slice from a garlic clove and placing it over the wart. Continue for a week and the wart should disappear.

- As a cure for nightmares, mince a clove or two of garlic into a bottle of red wine and take a glass each evening.

- Try rubbing foot corns with a cut clove of garlic every day until they disappear.

### What Is the Magic Ingredient?

The smelly part of garlic, allicin, has long been thought to be the magic ingredient of garlic. But it's now believed that the *by-products* of the breakdown of allicin—sulfides—provide the benefit, rather than the allicin itself.

When garlic is crushed or cut, allicin is released, together with its characteristic smell. Exactly the same process applies when garlic is chewed, and the allicin is released into the mouth.

As allicin breaks down it takes up oxygen, which assists its conversion into sulfur-rich chemicals. There are more than 70 of these sulfides, and most of these remain stable. In other words, their chemical form does not change. The fact that so many stable sulfides are produced may account for the wide range of illnesses that respond to garlic treatment, because each sulfide reacts in a different way to each disease.

## Garlic for Your Health

The next chapter examines the evidence that backs up many of the medical claims made in the case for eating garlic or taking it as a supplement. The rest of the book will address the problem of how best to use garlic to your benefit.

# 2

# Garlic for Your Health

## Garlic and Heart Disease

The heart is the body's most important muscle. Unlike every other muscle in the body, it never rests. It works nonstop, day and night, pumping blood into our lungs. In the lungs the blood picks up oxygen, which it carries to every single organ and nearly every tissue of the body. Meanwhile, oxygen-depleted blood is drawn back to the heart via the veins—and the cycle begins all over again.

If the heart ever stopped, we would be dead within minutes. But this vital organ relies, just as much as every other part of the body, on a supply of oxygen being fed through the coronary arteries. However, with age, most people's arteries begin to show the signs of wear and tear. By the age of 30 most of us will have suffered some degree of arteriosclerosis, which means that our arteries have thickened and developed lesions that hinder the flow of blood.

Arteriosclerosis can happen in any part of the body, but it's most dramatically noticed in the arteries around the heart. If the narrowing of a coronary artery exceeds a certain limit, the transport of blood and oxygen will be critically impeded. The result is a shortage of oxygen, particularly when demand for it is high, as for example when the heart beats fast during emotional stress or physical exercise. (We've all heard or read of people dying of "shock" or in the middle of running a marathon.) And the lack of blood and oxygen (ischemia, or hypoxia) is felt as angina pectoris—a pain in the heart, and often in the left arm or shoulder, accompanied by anxiety, fear, and breathlessness.

Angina pectoris is a warning sign that some dangerous narrowing has taken place in the vital arteries around the heart. If this is allowed to continue, there is a risk of suffering a heart attack, in which the lack of blood and oxygen is so severe that the whole or part of the heart muscle is starved of oxygen and the affected cells die.

Because about one-third of heart attacks happen without the early warning signs of angina, and death is therefore the first and last sign of the disease, it's critically important that we all take care of our hearts.

However healthy we may feel, it's always worth looking at our diet and lifestyle and improving them if we can.

The main risk factor for coronary heart disease is the balance of fats (lipids) in our blood. Some of these fats (high density lipoprotein, HDL) are healthy and help protect the heart. Others (low density lipoprotein, LDL) increase the risk of heart disease.

Ideally, you should have a low level of LDL and a high level of HDL. Imagine the HDL as a pint of raw milk with the LDL as the cream on the top. It's more important to know that this balance is right than to know what your total fat (or cholesterol) level is. Although you can now buy a DIY blood-cholesterol test over the counter from a pharmacist or a medical supplies store, only a doctor's full lipid test will tell you about your LDL:HDL ratio. So remember that while high levels of cholesterol *increase* your risk of developing heart disease, high levels of HDL actually *reduce* that risk.

A high LDL content in your blood increases your risk of heart disease by causing fatty deposits to stick to the walls of the artery, contributing to the process of arteriosclerosis. Studies have shown that this progression can be retarded by cholesterol reduction. Blood lipids are also affected by other factors, such as smoking and diabetes.

Garlic helps lower LDL levels without the side effects that may be felt with conventional lipid-lowering drugs. And, combined with a better diet and regular exercise (which will help your general health and well-being), garlic can bring cholesterol levels back into the normal range. It has the additional advantage of triggering antioxidant activity. This inhibits the process of oxidization of blood lipids, which makes them even more dangerous.

In Germany, practitioners of conventional medicine routinely prescribe garlic supplements for the treatment of arteriosclerosis. In Great Britain, these supplements used to be prescribable, but are no longer, owing to government intervention. And in the United States, garlic treatments are generally recommended only by alternative health practitioners, holistic healers, and the like.

However, there is evidence that garlic helps prevent coronary heart disease in various ways, by:

- Significantly lowering mildly elevated blood pressure

- Normalizing blood glucose levels in diabetic patients

- Improving blood flow by making blood more fluid, blood cells less sticky, and platelets less aggregable

- Influencing the blood-clotting system so that thromboses are less likely to form and more likely to be dissolved if they begin to form an obstruction

- Preventing irregular heartbeats and injury of the cells when there is a shortage of oxygen

- Limiting the ability of the cells in the vessel walls to grow, multiply, and form arteriosclerotic lesions

From his research into garlic and the heart, Professor Edzard Ernst, professor of complementary medicine at Exeter University in the U.K., has concluded that one would need to take an awful lot of synthetic drugs to obtain all the beneficial effects that garlic produces. He cites one study that compared garlic with bezafibrate, the most commonly prescribed lipid-lowering drug in the U.K. The results showed that patients in both groups had a 25 percent lowering of cholesterol levels, which means that garlic can be just as effective as the medication prescribed by your doctor—but without the side effects.

## Garlic and the Heart: The Evidence So Far

- In the early 1980s Professor Ernst studied 20 patients with high cholesterol levels and gave them either a cholesterol-lowering diet or the diet plus 600 mg. dried garlic powder per day. After just 12 days, levels of cholesterol, LDL, and triglyceride (another type of fat in the blood) fats were lower among the patients taking garlic.

- A recent study of 200 patients with elevated cholesterol levels compared garlic pills with a placebo and found that in those taking garlic the average decrease of cholesterol was 12 percent and the decrease of triglycerides was 17 percent.

- After a fatty meal the level of triglycerides tends to rise dramatically. Volunteers ate two test meals, each containing a minimum of 100 g. of butter. Before one meal, they were given 900 mg. of garlic powder. Before the other, no premedication was given. The rise in triglycerides was markedly attenuated after taking garlic.

- Professor Ernst also tested the effect of garlic when cholesterol was not high in the first place. The study, on normal volunteers, still showed a decrease in total cholesterol levels.

- Garlic has also been compared to a lipid-lowering drug, and has been found to be just as effective: patients in both test groups experienced a lowering of their cholesterol levels by 25 percent.

## Coping with a Heart Attack

### *David's Story*

David was just 37 years old when he woke suddenly at 5 a.m. with excruciating chest pains. Horrified, his wife Lynn telephoned their family doctor for help, and the doctor called 911 to summon an ambulance. But by the time help arrived, an hour after his first symptoms, David was too weak to move and the paramedics had to carry him out of the house on a stretcher while Lynn rushed their frightened children over to a neighbor's house.

In the emergency room doctors broke the news that David had suffered the classic symptoms of a heart attack. David comments:

> At the time I couldn't believe it. I didn't see myself as the heart-attack type at all. It was only when I took a really close look at my lifestyle that I realized how badly I'd let myself go. I'd become a complete slob. Although I had a physical job as a mechanical pipefitter, I had not taken any exercise since giving up amateur soccer four years earlier. I was also eating great big fried breakfasts and huge roast dinners every day, and I'd gained 42 pounds, which was enough to put me in the "obese" bracket.

David's children, James and Laura, were only 13 and 9 years old when he had his attack, and it was the fear of leaving them without a father and Lynn without a husband that spurred on his recovery.

"Another patient on my ward dropped dead in front of me," David says. "That was a chilling experience and I was determined not to let it happen to me.'"

The chance of suffering a second heart attack is highest during the first year after recovery, and, with this thought in mind, David did everything in his power to turn his health around.

He was out of bed within days, for, according to heart specialist Dr. Ian Baird, medical spokesperson for the British Heart Foundation, early mobility is to be greatly encouraged.

"People used to be kept in bed for weeks," says Dr. Baird, "but now we aim to get them up and used to taking a few steps as soon as possible."

Rehabilitation is an essential part of recovery and follows a four-stage plan, explains Dr. Baird.

During the week or so that patients are in the hospital they are counseled about what has happened and why, and told how they can help prevent a second attack. Then, two or three weeks after the heart attack, they'll come back to the hospital for an exercise test.

"They're asked to walk on a treadmill while an electrocardiogram measures the effect on the heart and assesses any changes," Dr. Baird says. "As well as giving the doctor a lot of very useful information, it is reassuring to the patient to know how much he can do without harming himself."

The second stage involves continued recovery and a course of mobilization at home, with a lot of support by way of therapist visits and visiting nurse calls. And, as Dr. Baird says:

> A patient will also be given medication to take. The most popular medicine is aspirin, which reduces

blood-clotting. But beta-blockers may also be given if high blood pressure or anxiety are problems.

Around this time a lot of heart patients start to worry about the stress that sexual activity will place on their heart, and many are also too embarrassed to ask for advice. What we generally say is that, as long as you can walk quickly up two flights of stairs without suffering discomfort or becoming breathless, you are safe to have sex. And this is usually only two to six weeks into recovery.

But it is a known fact that a sudden change in sexual partners could do more harm than good. So stick to your usual partner—and your usual sexual positions!

Some 6 to 12 weeks after the heart attack, patients recovering at home will still be having supervised exercise sessions with therapists and regular chats with a dietitian. They should now be regaining their confidence.

Finally, an outpatient review will be set up to see if any further investigations are necessary. Many patients are doing so well by this stage that they can safely return to work. The investigations, if required, will be noninvasive, and are most likely to involve an echocardiogram, which measures, with ultrasound equipment, the flow of blood being pumped by the heart. If the flow is greatly reduced, a treatment such as ACE inhibitors may be prescribed to combat narrowing of the blood vessels and prevent recurrent heart attacks.

"Twenty-five years ago one-third of all heart attack patients died," Dr. Baird says. "Now the figure is down to about 5 to 10 percent, and less than 3 percent for people under the age of 50."

Like many patients, David felt he was really achieving something on his rehabilitation program and he enjoyed reporting back to the hospital as he made continued progress with the changes to his diet and lifestyle:

> For 12 weeks I took supervised exercise at the hospital gym. Then I joined a local heart support group, and that was a fantastic help. We continued with the same kind of exercise routine, and I also made wonderful friends through the group.
>
> It is a myth that your life becomes restricted after a heart attack. There is still so much—if not more—to enjoy. But earlier this year I heard of a local woman who committed suicide because of heart problems. That was very sad because, had she known about our group, I'm sure we could have helped her.

David cut out all but the minimum of fatty foods from his diet and now makes sure the whole family eats a lot more fruit, vegetables, poultry, and fish. He adds:

> Lynn and I have also taken up a lot of walking—something the latest addition to our family, our dog Ben, thanks us for.
>
> I'm still taking a child's aspirin every day to keep my blood thin (after—not before—I shave, so that any nicks will clot quickly), but I feel great. The heart attack did me a favor, not a disservice. I've lost all that excess weight. I look and feel 100 percent better. And, to be honest, if I hadn't been

shocked into changing my lifestyle when I did, I'd hate to think what state I'd be in by now.

Swapping his daily dose of baby aspirin (usually 82 mg.) for a recommended garlic supplement would give David the same advantages without the drawbacks of aspirin that some people experience.

Regular use of aspirin can irritate the stomach lining, so avoid it if you have a history of stomach problems. You should also avoid it if you have a bleeding disorder, as aspirin can thin the blood and is often prescribed to slow blood-clotting. Some people, especially asthmatics, may also suffer an allergic reaction to aspirin. If you can safely take aspirin, the soluble variety is less likely to irritate your stomach—but seriously consider garlic as a safe alternative.

## Coping with Angina

### Jane's Story

At just 32, Jane found it hard to believe she could be a candidate for the heart disease angina. But everything she read on the disease seemed to describe her own symptoms to a Tee.

Since the birth of her daughter, Sarah, she'd had less time for exercise, and found the slightest exertion—running for a train, or walking any distance—brought on a strange icy sensation in her back, and, later, her arms. Jane says:

> When Sarah was nearly two, I was convinced I had angina, and my doctor referred me to a cardiologist

who confirmed the diagnosis. It didn't come as any surprise. By this time I was unable to walk even down the block or up the stairs without pausing for a rest.

A stress EKG (electrocardiogram) showed that the oxygen flow to Jane's heart during exercise was insufficient, and she was referred for an angiogram. Jane explains:

The doctor had to pass a catheter from my groin through the blood vessels to my heart. A dye was then passed through the tube, and an X-ray performed to show up any narrowings or blockages where the dye could not get through.

The result showed that, of Jane's three coronary arteries, only one was completely clear of blockage. Of the other two, one was 95 percent blocked, and the other 65 percent blocked. Her cardiologist explained the treatment options:

- For some patients in Jane's condition, drug treatment can increase blood supply to the heart, or reduce the work the heart has to do.

- Where drugs are unsuitable, a balloon angioplasty can widen the narrowed arteries and has the advantage of avoiding major surgery. But, for one in five patients, angina recurs within six months of this procedure.

- In the most serious cases, bypass surgery is recommended. This involves taking a piece of vein from elsewhere in the body (usually the leg) and using it to form a new, clear route to the heart that bypasses the blocked arteries.

"In my case the blockage was so severe that a bypass was the only option," Jane says. "It was a shock, but a relief too, because I knew it would cure my angina and give me a new start."

The operation took place the day before Jane's 34th birthday, and she was able to return home within a week. Jane says:

> The worst thing was not being able to pick Sarah up, but within six months Joe (my partner), Sarah, and I were all able to go on a lovely vacation and I felt as fit as a fiddle.
>
> The hospital ran an excellent rehabilitation program and it was a great confidence-booster to discover I could work up a sweat in the gym without any accompanying pain.
>
> I am no longer afraid of exercise, and I swim or do aerobics at least three times a week. I've also improved my diet and have given up all the cheese, chocolate, and butter I used to consume before becoming ill.
>
> I am closely monitored by the hospital, which helps. I know I'm fit, and Joe and I are even planning to have another child. I've talked to my cardiologist, obstetrician, and family physician, and they have all said they see no reason why I shouldn't have a normal, healthy pregnancy. So, with luck, Sarah will soon have a brother or sister!
>
> Had my condition not been diagnosed when it was, another pregnancy would have been out of the question. In fact, I would be lucky to have survived at all. I'm just relieved that I took the trouble to

worry about that weird sensation in my back and arms and to follow it up.

The benefits of garlic to the heart are indisputable, but what of the other health claims?

## Garlic and AIDS

At the time of writing there is no cure for AIDS (acquired immunodeficiency syndrome). So how can garlic help? It can be used, as shown in Chapter 3, to treat the many minor symptoms suffered by people with AIDS, such as genital herpes, recurrent fever, and candidiasis. But, of particular interest, some studies have suggested that HIV (the virus that's thought to cause AIDS) doesn't grow well in the presence of garlic, and patients' immune systems have also been strengthened after taking just one clove of garlic a day, either mashed in food or blended and disguised in a drink. However, more research needs to be done.

## Garlic and Blood Pressure

A "normal" blood pressure reading is around 120/80 (which the nurse taking it will pronounce as "120 over 80"). The first figure is the systolic, measuring the pressure inside the arteries the instant the heart beats. The second figure is the diastolic, measuring the pressure in the arteries when the heart is resting. If your systolic measurement is 140 or higher and the diastolic is 90 or higher, you have high blood pressure (hypertension).

Garlic can help stabilize high blood pressure, but you should take other steps too:

- Try to keep your weight within the right limits for your height.
- Don't eat too many fatty foods.
- Don't smoke.
- Drink alcohol in moderation.
- Try to avoid stress, and relax more.

> ### Garlic and High Blood Pressure: The Evidence So Far
>
> The *Journal of Hypertension* reported in 1997 that garlic powder tablets could reduce systolic blood pressure by 10 percent and diastolic blood pressure by 6 percent. The report went on to say that the potential blood-pressure lowering effect was of such significance that "stroke may be reduced by 30–40 percent and coronary heart disease by 20–25 percent."
>
> The authors, Professor Christopher Silagy and Dr. Andrew Neil, working at the Radcliffe Hospital in Oxford, U.K., looked at all the published data on garlic and blood pressure and conducted a review using strict guidelines to include only studies that had been properly designed and conducted. Overall, 415 subjects had been studied and they had all been treated with the same powdered garlic tablets (Kwai brand). The results showed that both systolic and diastolic blood pressure were significantly reduced.

Regular exercise and a salt-free diet also help. If you find your food tasteless without salt, as an alternative use garlic powder, or try some of the food-enhancer mixes available in supermarkets or health food stores.

Dr. F. G. Piotrowski of the University of Geneva, Switzerland, found, in 1948, that the sulfur compounds in garlic calm the nerves. This, combined with the effects I've already mentioned, of strengthening the heart and dilating restricted blood vessels, helps to bring blood pressure down. There's anecdotal evidence that garlic works even better in lowering high blood pressure when it's combined with watercress, so try putting both in your daily salad (see the recipes in Chapter 5).

## Garlic and Cancer

Researchers are becoming very excited at the prospect that garlic may hinder the growth of cancerous tumors. In test tubes, garlic has been shown to kill bacteria, viruses, and fungi and to stimulate the immune system, which could ultimately render it useful in treating cancer and perhaps other diseases as well.

Researchers in Pennsylvania have shown that, by injecting a compound called diallyl disulfide (formed when raw garlic is cut or crushed), tumors can be reduced by half and that a further compound (S-Allylcysteine) can stop cancer-causing agents from binding to human breast cells. But a report in the *British Journal of Cancer* in 1993 concluded that evidence from laboratory experiments and population surveys is presently not conclusive as to the preventative activity of garlic. However, the available evidence warrants further research into the possible role of garlic in the prevention of cancer in humans.

## Garlic and Circulation

Evidence is accumulating that garlic and garlic supplements may help to improve circulation. By making your blood less likely to clot, garlic can reduce blood-platelet aggregation. (That is, because your blood becomes slightly thinner, the platelets are prevented from sticking together and clogging your arteries.) It has also been reported that garlic will reduce blood thickening. In one study that looked at capillary blood flow in the nail folds of the hand, garlic increased blood flow by 55 percent, and in patients who had peripheral arterial occlusive disease (partially clotted arteries, particularly in the legs) garlic tablets slightly improved walking distance.

About 70 different sulfur compounds are released via the breakdown of allicin in a cut clove or crushed clove of garlic, and one of these compounds—ajoene—possesses antithrombotic (anticlotting) properties and has been proved to have a significant antiplatelet effect.

In a double-blind placebo controlled study where neither the patient nor the investigator knew whether the patient was taking a placebo drug or a Kwai-brand garlic tablet, spontaneous thrombocyte aggregation disappeared (that is, the blood stopped sticking together), microcirculation to the skin increased by 47 percent, and both blood pressure and blood glucose levels were decreased in those taking garlic.

## Coping with Thrombosis

### Jacqueline's Story

When Jacqueline was put on HRT (hormone replacement therapy) after being plunged into an early menopause at the age of 31, she was aware that the treatment carried a remote risk of causing the blood-clotting disorder deep vein thrombosis.

"Four out of every thousand women using HRT develop problems," says Jacqueline, now 37. "But being younger than the average menopausal woman, and having a healthy lifestyle, I really didn't consider myself a candidate."

After years of trouble with long and heavy periods and with painful endometriosis, Jacqueline had been given a total hysterectomy, which included the removal of her ovaries. Her HRT patches had been prescribed to replace the hormones her body was no longer able to produce on its own.

She had been told that the usual warning sign of thrombosis is a deep pain in the back of the calf, but she became alarmed when, a year after starting the HRT, she suddenly developed a heavy and throbbing sensation in her breast. "It was similar to the feeling I remembered from when my milk came in after the births of my three children, Leanne, 18, Lorraine, 16, and Ashley, 7," Jacqueline says.

> Two days later, I was in the shower when I saw an angry red lump and a raised vein on my breast. I was beside myself with worry and went straight to my doctor, who immediately recognized it as thrombosis and took me off the HRT.

She prescribed aspirin to thin the blood and break down the clot. The lump vanished without a trace within a week, and there was no need for me to go into the hospital. Unfortunately, my doctor thinks it's now better for me to stay off HRT, and that means that, even six years on, I have to put up with horrible menopausal symptoms, and I am worried that I am at risk of developing osteoporosis, which affects a lot of postmenopausal women.

But I consider myself very lucky that the clot was in such an obvious place. My grandmother died of deep vein thrombosis at the age of 53. And, because I work out regularly at the gym, I may have mistaken the pain for muscle strain if it had been in my calf.

Dr. Philip Hannaford of the Royal College of General Practitioners in Great Britain says it's not unusual for women on HRT or the Pill to worry that they won't recognize the symptoms of thrombosis in the calf. He explains:

The tell-tale sign is a distinctive pain, deep in the calf, accompanied by a hot swelling and hardening of the area. Stretching the back of the leg by pulling your toes towards your knees will increase the pain, but your doctor will be able to tell you whether this is due to thrombosis or straightforward muscle strain.

Because a clot in the calf is not as clearly visible as Jacqueline's was, you may well be referred to a hospital or clinic where the diagnosis can be confirmed, using a dye test (a venogram) or an ultrasound scan.

You'd normally be taken off the Pill or HRT and may be prescribed anticoagulant drugs or aspirin for a few months, to break down any clotting while the cause of the thrombosis (say, a genetic link) is investigated.

Some women go back on the Pill or HRT without problems. But, after one scare, most are reluctant to do so. If you do continue treatment, your doctor would want to monitor you very closely and probably prescribe longer-term anticoagulants to minimize the risk. You may even be given a form of HRT containing a synthetic alternative to estrogen, because it's the estrogen and the way it reacts with progesterone that is thought to increase the blood's clotting capability in some women.

> **DEEP VEIN THROMBOSIS** is caused by a combination of sluggish blood flow and some condition that increases the blood's natural tendency to clot. The Pill (especially the lower estrogen "third generation" brands) and HRT appear to increase clotting in some women, but the risk to users remains extremely low. Only one in 10,000 Pill-users, and four out of every 1,000 women on HRT, will develop the condition. And, among them, only one or two women will die, in the very unusual situation where a blood clot has traveled symptomlessly to the lung.
> Any unusual pains or swellings should be reported to your doctor. Chest pain and breathlessness may be the only warning signs of a clot in your lung, and should be taken very seriously.

"Thrombosis is extremely rare, and usually mild and easily treated," says Dr. Hannaford. "But whatever your concerns or symptoms, you have the right to discuss them with your family doctor, and no sensible doctor will feel you are wasting his or her time by asking for reassurance."

## Garlic and Diabetes

Whether garlic can increase insulin secretion is unclear, but a study has shown an 11 percent reduction in blood glucose in patients taking garlic tablets. As diabetics tend to be at greater risk of problems with high blood pressure, cholesterol, and circulation, some doctors have said that taking a garlic supplement is a sensible course of action for such patients.

# 3

# Garlic as a Remedy for Common Ailments

BECAUSE OF ITS ANTIBACTERIAL and antifungal properties, garlic has traditionally been used to treat everything from acne to toothache. Although it's a messy, smelly, and strong-tasting preparation (the main reasons why so many of us have turned to over-the-counter medicines!), interest in this natural medicine is being revived.

The medical herbalist Dian Dincin Buchman says garlic is one of her favorite herbs:

> If garlic wasn't so cheap we would treasure it as if it were pure gold. It adds valuable natural cleansing, infection-fighting chemicals to the daily diet, and can be made into a vinegar tincture for antiseptic use, a

syrup to control asthma, and an oil for internal and external use. Garlic draws out pain, calms nerves, helps resist colds. It's nothing short of fantastic and its use can be traced to centuries of use among many cultures.

Here are some of the many ways in which naturopaths, holistic healers, and herbalists use garlic to treat common ailments.

### ACNE

Acne spots develop when hair follicles are blocked with sebum, the oily substance secreted by the sebaceous glands beneath the skin. It's most common in puberty, when a change in hormone levels takes place and more sebum is secreted. Usually this hormonal activity settles down after adolescence, and an adult's complexion will be relatively blemish-free. A sudden return to acne in adulthood is often a sign of a hormone imbalance.

Doctors say there's no evidence that diet plays any part in causing acne. Surprisingly, although most of us connect chocolate with blemishes, it actually has no effect on the skin. However, stress can be a contributory factor, and you're more likely to develop acne when you're under stress.

Doctors normally recommend that patients start off trying to clear their acne by using topical lotions such as antibiotic or sulfur-containing creams. If these fail, long-term treatment with oral antibiotic drugs may be recommended, but these can set up other health problems such as thrush (candidiasis—see page 34) and a low immune system.

If the sufferer (usually a teenager) can bear it, and can go into hibernation for a few days, ready to emerge as a transformed and spotless beauty, she or he can either make a face mask using three chopped cloves of garlic mixed with a spoonful of honey and a tablespoon of kaolin powder, or refrigerate a mixture of chopped garlic (about four cloves) with 8 fl. oz. of surgical spirit, and apply it directly to the pimples. In both cases, care should be taken to avoid getting the mixture in the eyes, as it will sting.

## ANEMIA

The condition called anemia (a lack of hemoglobin in the blood) is caused when there's not enough iron in the body to allow its production, although inadequate vitamin C, B vitamins, protein, iodine, copper, and cobalt can also contribute to the problem. Garlic in your diet increases the absorption of B vitamins, especially vitamin $B_1$, and it also contains copper, which, together with vitamin C (also in garlic), greatly improves iron assimilation.

## ANIMAL BITES

Garlic water and a garlic poultice (see page 50) can help to clean up a superficial wound, since garlic acts as a natural antiseptic and antibacterial cleaner.

## ARTHRITIS

Drinking garlic tea (see page 50) can help soothe aching joints. Some people are reported to sip the tea with their feet up and crushed garlic rubbed into their soles! Garlic can also be used as a hot liniment that's massaged into the joints.

## ASTHMA

This is a serious condition, so don't attempt to treat it without professional help and supervision. However, the combination of honey and garlic has been known to stem attacks. Use the remedy (one crushed clove of garlic mixed with a tablespoon of raw honey) at the first sign of onset.

Dian Dincin Buchman recommends the following recipe, which has been handed down through her family:

| | |
|---|---|
| 8 oz. peeled garlic | ½ pint glycerin |
| Equal amounts of vinegar and distilled water to cover the garlic | ½ lb. honey |

Put the peeled garlic, water, and vinegar in a jar with a tight-fitting lid and shake it well. Store it for four days in a cool place, shaking it once or twice a day. Then add the glycerin, shake again, and leave it to stand for another day. Finally, strain the liquid, blend it with the honey, and store in a cool place.

Take one teaspoon (with water if desired) every 15 minutes until the asthma attack is under control, and then once every two to three hours.

## ATHLETE'S FOOT

If the webs between your fourth and fifth (little) toes are itchy, sore, and cracked, you probably have athlete's foot. The good news is that it's easily treated—and you can prevent reinfection, too.

Athlete's foot is usually caused by the fungal infection tinea pedis, but can also be caused by bacteria. It's spread in changing rooms and public shower areas, so take extra precautions to clean and dry your feet scrupulously—especially between your toes—after going to the gym or using other athletic facilities and swimming pools.

Infection is rare in young children, and is usually associated with sweaty feet and shoes. If you go barefoot a lot of the time, you're less likely to suffer.

Athlete's foot can clear up without medication, and drying your feet, especially in between your toes, will help. You should also try to wear cotton socks and sandals.

If you don't fancy the idea of antifungal creams (the usual treatment for athlete's foot), try soaking the affected area in cider vinegar, and then drying it with arrowroot powder and applying tea tree oil, which has antifungal qualities.

- *Garlic remedy:* Look after your feet as above, and rub one crushed clove of garlic into the affected area daily. Leave for half an hour before you rinse off. By the end of the week, you should be free of infection.

## BLISTERS

Smearing a blister with the oil squeezed out of a commercial garlic "pearle" is reported to have more effect than traditional over-the-counter remedies.

## BOILS

Rub a garlic and honey mixture (as prescribed for asthma—see page 32) into an infected boil to bring relief.

## BRONCHITIS

Drink garlic tea to ease congestion in your chest, and avoid dairy products for the duration of your cough as these will exacerbate it.

## BURNS

Remove the heat from a minor burn by soaking the area in cold (not iced) water. Then rub the oil from a garlic pearle into the burn. However, if the burn shows any signs of blistering or splitting, don't rub oil into it, as it will seal in the heat and aggravate the injury.

## CANDIDIASIS (THRUSH)

Also known as thrush or moniliasis, candidiasis is an infection caused by the fungus *candida albicans*. It most commonly affects the vagina but also affects other areas of mucous membrane, such as inside the mouth, or moist skin. Vaginal candidiasis may cause a thick, white, cottage cheese–like discharge as well as vaginal itching and irritation.

The fungus that causes candidiasis is normally present in the mouth and the vagina, but is kept under control by the bacteria usually present in these organs. A course of antibiotics may destroy too many of the bacteria, allowing the fungus to multiply. Or the growth of the fungus may become excessive due to hormonal changes—typically, those that take place in pregnancy.

The infection is much more common in women than in men, although it can be passed between partners during intercourse. The infection may spread from the genitals or mouth to other moist areas of the body. It can also affect the gastrointestinal tract, especially in people who have impaired immune systems.

In infants, candidiasis sometimes occurs in conjunction with diaper rash.

Orthodox treatment is with antifungal drugs, usually prescribed in the form of vaginal suppositories or creams. Your sexual partner should be treated at the same time to prevent reinfection.

- *Garlic remedy:* Caroline Clayton, author of *Coping with Thrush* (Sheldon Press), recommends inserting garlic cloves, sliced in half and wrapped in gauze, directly into the vagina. Alternatively, she offers the following garlic treatments, to be used as a vaginal douche, and says garlic is useful when more than one infection is present in the vagina at any one time.

Put eight cloves of garlic in a jar with about ½ pint of white, sugarless vinegar. Leave this by an open window for about two days, until the oil of the garlic has been released. Use a tablespoon of this solution in 1 pint of water. Use twice a day for a week.

Or:

Boil 1 pint of water with a peeled and chopped clove of garlic for about 15 minutes, strain and leave to cool. Use twice a day for a week.

## CHILBLAINS

Applying garlic oil to the affected area will help local irritation. Because chilblains usually accompany a circulatory problem, it's a good idea to add garlic to your diet too, to improve your circulation.

## COLDS AND FLU

Garlic won't cure a cold or flu, because these are viral infections and untreatable with antibiotics, but it can alleviate symptoms. Try a steam inhalation of garlic in water to clear your sinuses. A drink of garlic crushed into warm milk is also recommended by Dr. Reg Saynor, a consulting lipidologist who has studied garlic.

## COLD SORES

Strictly for those with a sense of humor as well as a problem with cold sores, the following remedy is reported to bring fast relief: crush a clove of garlic and hold it in place on the sore with a bandage.

## CONSTIPATION

Hippocrates recommended garlic for constipation, as it stimulates the peristaltic motion of the intestinal walls to produce a bowel movement.

## CYSTITIS

If you suffer with cystitis, you're not alone: it's one of the most common complaints women experience. The symptoms—burning pain on urination, an urge to urinate frequently, and dark, strong-smelling urine—progress rapidly. Within an hour of first realizing an attack is starting, you can be in severe pain. So act quickly to make yourself more comfortable.

The cause is usually bacterial. *E. coli*, which lives happily in the bowel, wreaks havoc in the bladder. But bruising of the urethra (sometimes through having frequent sex, when it's known as "honeymoon cystitis") can cause the same painful symptoms without any infection.

You may want to avoid passing water because of the pain it causes, and be tempted to drink as little as possible. Don't give in to the temptation. Instead, you should drink like a fish, and go to the bathroom as often as you can, to stem the multiplication of the bacteria and flush out the bladder.

- Drink large quantities of alkaline fluids. Several pints of water an hour, with a teaspoonful of bicarbonate of soda to every pint, or lemon barley water are ideal.

- If you're a recurrent sufferer and use the diaphragm as your contraceptive method, you should consider another form of birth control.

- Build up your immune system with plenty of vitamin C. Recurrent cystitis is a sign that your body is slow to fight infection.

- Don't drink tea or coffee last thing at night, as they make an attack more likely. Water is best.

- To prevent the bacteria's getting into the urethra from the bowel during intercourse, empty your bladder before and after sex. Also make sure you wipe "front to back" when you've been to the toilet. Good hygiene is essential to avoid repeated attacks.

Your doctor will need to test your urine so that she can prescribe the correct antibiotic. If antibiotics give you thrush, try natural (unsweetened) cranberry juice, which prevents the bacteria from clinging to the lining of the bladder and the urethra.

- *Garlic remedy:* Add garlic to your diet or take it as a supplement to ward off infection, and drink garlic tea (see page 50) throughout the day when you are infected.

**DIARRHEA**

The problem should clear up on its own, but you may need to help it along the way. If you still have an appetite, try to eat as little as possible, especially in the way of rich foods, and make sure you drink plenty of water. If you're abroad, this must be pure—boiled and then cooled—water. If you can buy bottled mineral water, make sure it's a brand you are familiar with, and check that the seal at the top of the bottle hasn't been broken, so you know it's the genuine article.

Over-the-counter antidiarrheal tablets will slow the upset down if your diarrhea is getting out of hand, and rehydration salts, added to your water, will speed up recovery. Especially for babies and young children, a preparation such as Pedialyte is essential to the first-aid kit when you are traveling abroad. Infants dehydrate much more rapidly than adults, and these salts will provide them with the minerals needed to rebalance their system.

Eating raw garlic daily is recommended for travelers who want to avoid getting "the runs," because the parasites or bacteria that cause the problem will be less likely to survive. But garlic capsules can also help clear up an attack that has started. Joan and Lydia Wilen, authors of *Garlic—Nature's Super Healer* (Prentice Hall), advise taking one capsule twice a day for a mild attack, two capsules three times a day if it's moderate, or two capsules four times a day if it's severe.

## DIGESTIVE PROBLEMS

Garlic as an ingredient of your meals will help prevent indigestion before it starts, as it helps stimulate the secretion of digestive enzymes and relieves problems such as gas and heartburn.

## EARACHE

Squeeze the oil from a punctured garlic pearle into your ear and plug it with a cotton ball or two.

## FATIGUE

If you're tired all the time, you should see your family doctor to find out what's causing your fatigue. But if you're just feeling drowsy—the "Why can't I wake up today?" syndrome—cut open a clove of garlic and breathe in the smell, or take a few deep breaths from a punctured garlic pearle.

## GUM PROBLEMS

If your gums are sore and swollen, you should get them checked out by your dental hygienist, as you could have an infection caused by excess plaque. Garlic is also an ancient remedy for clearing up gum infections. But if you eat it raw it can burn your gums in the process, so capsules are best. Take two capsules every four hours for three days. (And call for that hygienist's appointment!)

## HANGOVERS

Inebriated laboratory animals have recovered quickly from alcohol poisoning with garlic treatment, according to Japanese scientists, and the alcohol has cleared from their blood faster than if it had been left to shift at its natural pace. Drinking the garlic-rich Mediterranean soup gazpacho when you're hung over (see page 81) has also been recommended.

## HAY FEVER

The condition known as hay fever (or seasonal allergic rhinitis) is an allergy to tree and grass pollens, molds, and spores. The allergy causes inflammation in the nose, making it feel itchy and blocked up. Sufferers sneeze a lot, their eyes itch and water, and they can sometimes suffer irritation in the mouth and ears, together with listlessness, depression, and poor concentration.

At the beginning of the hay-fever season a pollen count of 50 will trigger a reaction in most sufferers. Later in the season, when your nose is already inflamed and irritated, a lower pollen count may have the same effect.

To a certain extent you can avoid the conditions most likely to cause a bad reaction:

- Don't sit outside in the early evening, when the pollen count is at its highest.

- Keep your bedroom windows shut at night, and consider adding an air-cleaning unit to your sleeping room.

- Wear sunglasses to prevent pollen entering your eyes.

- Take seaside rather than country vacations, as the air by the coast is clear of pollen.

Avoiding the triggers will help in your battle against hay fever, but you'll probably also need one or more of the following treatments:

- *Antihistamines* (e.g., Benadryl, Dimetane, Seldane, and Claritin) will stop sneezing, but don't relieve congestion.

- *Intranasal corticosteroid sprays* (such as Aeroabid, Azmacort, and Dexacort) work on the site of the inflammation and prevent the nasal passages from swelling almost shut. They should be used from the very beginning of the hay-fever season, as they are largely a preventative treatment.

If you are taking any other medication, consult with your doctor or pharmacist before starting on a hay-fever treatment, as you may run the risk of a reaction if the drugs are used together.

♦ *Garlic remedy:* Mix one crushed clove of garlic with ¼ cup of hot water, allow to cool, and strain into a nose- or eye-drop bottle (available at any drugstore). Use as a nose-dropper, applying ten drops to each nostril three times a day for three days.

## HEADACHE

Garlic increases the body's absorption of vitamin $B_1$ (thiamin). This is vital to nerve health, and lack of it may contribute to headaches. Hot and cold garlic footbaths are reputed to help clear headaches. But do be careful not to take too much garlic if you're prone to headaches, as garlic has also been known to cause them.

## HEMORRHOIDS (PILES)

Using garlic (one clove at a time, once a day only, after a bowel movement) as a suppository will help disinfect the area and bring down the swelling that accompanies piles.

## HERPES

Eating garlic is supposed to hold back outbreaks of both genital and oral herpes. You can also apply a garlic poultice to a herpes sore to relieve it (see page 50).

## IMPOTENCE

Many men have, at some time or other, found themselves in the situation where they can't sustain an erection long enough to have sex, or can't achieve an erection suitable for penetration. It may be that the man has had too much alcohol, is tired, or simply isn't sufficiently attracted to his partner.

An occasional episode like this is normal in any man's sex life, and as long as they occur infrequently, there's no need to worry. But when impotence becomes a regular problem, it can wreak havoc in a couple's sex life.

Impotence, or "erectile difficulty," often occurs as a result of a combination of factors, but there's nearly always a psychological element involved.

If a man can't, under any circumstances, achieve an erection, then it's possible that he has a physical problem that needs to be treated. Anyone suffering from impotence will be given a medical checkup to pinpoint or rule out any illness. However, even when the basic cause is medical, the psychological side should also be looked at. Stress at work or in the relationship itself can cause a man to become impotent. So can anxiety about sexual performance, as can deep-seated feelings of guilt about sex.

If the problem is physical, the sufferer may be offered injections that he can use to induce an erection. These involve injecting a chemical substance into the blood tissues of the penis. But they have disadvantages, and some men find it difficult to get their erect penis back into a normal "resting" position. An erection that lasts a few hours may need to be aspirated by a doctor to bring it back down.

If the problem is not entirely a physical one, the sufferer may be referred to a sex therapist or counselor who will help him, preferably working with his partner too, to overcome the emotional problems behind his impotence.

- *Garlic remedy:* The French folk herbalist Maurice Messegue recommended that his patients massage their coccyx (the "tailbone" area) with crushed garlic, using a circular motion, for about ten minutes every day, a treatment that had a 40 percent success rate.

## INSECT BITES

*Six tips for dealing with insect bites and stings:*

1. Put cold packs on the inflamed area to soothe the skin.

2. Use a slice of raw onion as a poultice to draw out any poisonous toxins from the sting.

3. Dab vinegar onto wasp stings to reduce inflammation, but use an alkaline solution such as baking soda mixed with water for bee stings.

4. Eat plenty of garlic *before* you get stung, as it acts as a natural insect repellent.

5. Don't rub or irritate the inflamed area.

6. Scratch a bee stinger out of your skin instead of pulling it.

> ♦ *Garlic remedy:* In parts of the Middle East a clove of garlic is chewed and mixed with one's own saliva, and then rubbed on to the bite.

## MASTITIS

This condition affects many breastfeeding women, and is one of the disadvantages of breastfeeding, although the condition usually doesn't last too long, providing you're quick to recognize the symptoms and get the treatment you need.

The hormonal changes that occur during lactation will encourage the mastitis. (This is also seen in newborn babies. Their breasts can develop mastitis, regardless of the baby's sex, because they are so rich in their mother's hormone in the days following birth.)

Infectious mastitis is uncommon and more likely to happen when you're still in the hospital after the birth of your baby. The infection, which may be carried by the baby's nose, is passed into your breast via a cracked nipple. If infection is diagnosed, you may be advised to express your milk (using a breast pump) until it has cleared up, but after that there's is no reason why you shouldn't resume breastfeeding.

Noninfectious-mastitis occurs when a duct becomes blocked. You may feel hot and shivery, as if you're getting the flu, and your breast will feel very hot and tender and particularly painful when you feed your baby. However, it's important to persevere with feeding when the flow of milk is not obviously infected, because the baby's energetic suckling is positively beneficial in allowing congestion—and hence the inflammation of mastitis—to settle. You'll probably also need to take antibiotics to speed up the process.

Very occasionally, the infection will be so bad that an abscess will form, and this will need lancing to allow the infection to drain. In this case, antibiotics on their own will not be effective, and they may make matters worse: the treated abscess is in a germ-free state, but local swelling and scar tissue can continue to form.

Fortunately, it's now very rare for mastitis to reach abscess stage. Indeed, thanks to the careful teaching of modern midwives and birthing clinics and coaches, mastitis is far less common than it was even 40 years ago.

- *Garlic remedy:* Follow your doctor's advice, but also consider taking Lalitha Thomas's Enhanced Garlic Formula (see page 49).

## MORNING SICKNESS

Vomiting in pregnancy is usually called morning sickness, although pregnant women can be sick at any time of day and it can vary from mild nausea to frequent vomiting. It normally clears up once the placenta has taken over hormone production, around 12–14 weeks, but severe vomiting is cause for concern and needs treatment.

To alleviate normal pregnancy sickness:

- Try to have a cup of tea (not coffee) and a plain cookie or cracker before even getting out of bed.

- Eat small, frequent meals.

- Suck crystalized ginger root, or take some dried ginger powder mixed with honey.

Ginger is an excellent cure for nausea (remember the ginger-ale your mother gave you as a child?) and works wonders for morning sickness as well. If you want the benefits of ginger but can't stomach the taste of it, try taking capsules of dried ginger or ginger oil.

- *Garlic remedy:* Eat garlic to help the absorption of vitamin $B_1$ (thiamin), which helps relieve morning sickness.

## PMS

Almost all women suffer, sooner or later, from some sort of problem associated with premenstrual syndrome, or PMS. Some symptoms are emotional and psychological (e.g., anxiety, confusion, disturbed sleep). Others are behavioral (e.g., clumsiness and violent behavior), or physical (e.g., food cravings, breast tenderness, acne, headaches).

Some women control their symptoms with the help of vitamin $B_6$ (although high doses can cause nerve poisoning), evening primrose oil, tranquilizers, or an improved diet. Others need more drastic hormone treatment. Natural progesterone can be given in the form of a suppository or an injection. Injections tend to be reserved for the most severe cases, where the doctor is sure the PMS is brought on by lack of the "calming" hormone progesterone.

- *Garlic remedy:* Eat garlic to help the absorption of vitamin $B_6$.

### RINGWORM

This is the name given to certain types of fungal skin infections marked by ring-shaped reddened, scaly, or blistery patches on the skin. Its medical name is tinea, which covers a range of ringworm infections on the skin, hair, and nails.

The appearance and the symptoms of the tinea vary according to the site. The most common type is tinea pedis (athlete's foot—see page 32), which causes cracking and itching between the toes. Tinea corporis (ringworm of the body) is characterized by itchy patches on the body. These are usually circular with a prominent edge. Tinea cruris (jock itch) produces a reddened, itchy area spreading from the genitals outward over the inside of the thigh. This form of ringworm is more common among men.

Ringworm infections are often associated with lack of hygiene, and are therefore more common in areas where living conditions are poor or squalid, or in rural areas, where there's greater exposure to animals.

The fungi that cause the infections can be caught from another person, from an animal, from soil, from the floors of showers and locker rooms, or even from household objects such as chairs or carpets.

The fungus spreads by means of tiny spores that can be carried in the air. There are over 100,000 different species of fungi worldwide. Most are either harmless or positively beneficial to human health, like the yeasts used for brewing and baking. A few form colonies on the skin, leading to varying degrees of ringworm.

Ringworm tends to occur on the feet (athlete's foot) or genitals (jock itch), where conditions are moist and allow the fungus to thrive. Humid, hot weather conditions, and sweaty clothes are likely to be responsible for a sustained attack elsewhere on the body.

A doctor or dermatologist will usually diagnose ringworm from its appearance, but the diagnosis should be confirmed and the type of fungus identified by taking a culture from the skin and sending it to be developed in the special conditions of a laboratory.

For most types of ringworm, treatment is by means of antifungal drugs in the form of skin creams, lotions, or ointments. However, for widespread infections, or those affecting the hair or nails, an antifungal drug in tablet form may be necessary.

The patient may be advised to continue treatment for some time after the symptoms have subsided to prevent further recurrence, but treatment should normally be completed within four to six weeks.

- *Garlic remedy:* Mix two minced cloves of garlic with the oil from three vitamin E capsules and rub onto the ringworm patch three times a day.

## SCIATICA

The condition called sciatica is a pain that radiates along the sciatic nerve, usually affecting the buttock and thigh, but sometimes extending to the leg and foot. It's often caused by a prolapsed disc pressing on a spinal root of the nerve, and treatment is directed toward the cause of the pain. Analgesic drugs (painkillers) are traditionally prescribed, but doctors in ancient Rome treated sciatica by massaging the painful area with equal parts of olive oil and eucalyptus oil, and having the patient eat a raw clove of garlic daily. A garlic milk drink (two cloves of garlic, peeled and minced into half a cup of milk) taken daily for two weeks is also reported to bring relief.

## SINUSITIS

See the garlic nose-drop remedy used for hay fever (page 39).

## SORE THROAT

A sore throat is usually caused by an infection, and, as garlic is a natural antibiotic, it helps tremendously to eat at least two raw cloves of garlic every day. Garlic tea can also be used as a gargle and as a drink (see page 50).

## SUNBURN

Getting sunburned can ruin a vacation, as well as causing long-term skin damage. It's most likely to happen during the first few days, when your skin hasn't had a chance to build up its protective brown melanin, but prolonged exposure to the sun without a suitable sunscreen can result in damage at any time, so it's best not to take any risks.

*Five ways to ease sunburn:*
If your skin begins to redden or feels sore:
1. Stay out of the sun (wear wide-brimmed hats and long sleeves if you must venture outdoors).
2. Take a cool bath or shower and apply cool compresses.
3. Use a soothing lotion, such as aloe vera gel, to relieve discomfort and cool your skin.
4. Drink plenty of mineral water or soft drinks, and rest. Avoid alcohol, which could cause further dehydration.
5. Seek medical advice for skin that's badly burned or blistering, or if the person seems to be ill.

- *Garlic remedy:* Cool your skin with a wash cloth soaked in chilled garlic tea (see below), but don't let it get near your eyes, as it will sting.

### TOOTHACHE
Place a whole peeled clove of garlic directly on the aching tooth and keep it there for an hour.

# Remedies

### LALITHA THOMAS' ENHANCED GARLIC FORMULA
1 part garlic powder
¼ part cayenne powder
1 part powdered calcium ascorbate
Store in an airtight container in a cool dry place.

## GARLIC WATER

For internal use, crush one or two cloves of garlic into each quart of water. For external use, a ratio of one clove to a half a pint of water is fine.

## GARLIC POULTICE

Put crushed garlic in a piece of gauze or cheesecloth and hold in place with a tape or bandage. Put a hot, wet towel over it to keep it warm and moist. If your skin is sensitive, apply a little olive oil to the area before using the poultice.

## GARLIC TEA

Heat water just until it starts to bubble, but not yet boiling (as you don't want to boil away its beneficial properties!), and add ¼ teaspoon of garlic powder to each cup that you make. Drink warm, or cool for later use.

# 4

# Good Health and Garlic

As with any nutritious food or supplement, there's no point in adding garlic to your diet with the intention of improving your health if you continue to do other things that are bad for you. So, if you're serious about using garlic for its health properties, and not just to add flavor to your cooking, you should also look at the following:

## Your Diet

### FATS AND HEART DISEASE

Heart disease claims 740,000 lives in the United States each year, and it's estimated that at least 13,900,000 more people have evidence of heart disease.

The most common form in adults is coronary heart disease, which occurs when the arteries bringing oxygen-rich blood to your heart get "clogged up" (see Chapter 2).

The clogging-up (or coating) process is cumulative. It starts in childhood and is caused by the fatty foods in our diet, which can increase our blood-cholesterol levels and leave us with more than we need. The body can't always dispose of its surplus blood cholesterol, so it deposits it in the arteries, causing them to narrow or clog up.

Although there are often other factors involved in heart disease (notably being overweight, smoking, not getting enough exercise, and the genes you were born with), it's important to reduce the risk by cutting down on the fats in your diet.

> ## If my arteries are already blocked up, what difference will it make if I change my diet now?
>
> The foundations of heart disease are mostly laid in your teens and early adult life, but you may have no symptoms until middle or old age. Even if your arteries have already started to narrow, your chances of developing heart disease will be considerably reduced if you adopt an "anticoronary" lifestyle. This may involve giving up smoking, starting a course of regular exercise, *and* changing your diet.
>
> In addition to a lower-fat diet, certain foods high in soluble fiber, such as legumes (peas, beans, lentils, and the like), fruit, and oats, can significantly help to reduce the amount of cholesterol in your blood.

- Angina occurs when your heart doesn't receive enough oxygen. An attack is often triggered by exercise or emotional stress, which are times when your heart needs extra oxygen.

- A heart attack occurs if the coronary artery becomes completely blocked, either because of the clogging process or if a blood clot forms.

## GOOD AND BAD FATS

We need a small amount of fat in our diet to provide us with certain vitamins, and also to make our food more tasty. However, there are *beneficial* fats and then there are *harmful* fats, and it's the bad ones we should be getting rid of.

The difference between "good" and "bad" fats is in the chemical structure of the fatty acids that make them up. Fatty acids are long chains of carbon atoms joined by a chemical bond, which may be either double or single.

It's the fatty acids with no double bonds that are saturates. Where there's only one double bond, it's known as a monounsaturated fat, and where there are two or more, the fatty acid is called polyunsaturated.

Most fats are made up of a mixture of many fatty acids. For example, the fat in butter is 63 percent saturated, 3 percent polyunsaturated, and 34 percent monounsaturated fatty acids. So when you hear that butter is a "saturated fat," what it really means is that it's higher in saturated fat than in any other kind.

Saturated fats are bad for us because high levels of them in the blood block and damage the arteries and impede blood circulation, increasing the risk of cardiovascular disease. (If you need a visual reminder of how this works, look at the grease congealed in the frying pan after you've cooked a hamburger or a fatty steak.)

Most of us are now aware of the risks of a very high-fat diet, and over the last 15 years many of us have dramatically changed the way we eat. Gone from most breakfast tables is the traditional fried eggs with bacon.

Nevertheless, there's still a lot of confusion about why polyunsaturated fats are good for us. In fact, they make the blood less "sticky," which prevents it from attaching itself to arterial walls and causing blockages. Hence their beneficial effect on your health—unless you eat so much of them that your weight becomes a health problem!

Saturated fat is also thought to be a factor in the level of cholesterol in the blood.

Cholesterol can originate in two ways:

1. Blood (serum) cholesterol is manufactured by the liver and is an essential part of all healthy cells. The liver makes enough cholesterol for our needs, and a high level of saturated fat in our diet can make the liver produce more cholesterol than is needed by the body.

2. Dietary cholesterol is cholesterol found in foods. Animal foods that are high in saturated fat are also high in cholesterol, and some low-fat foods also contain high levels. You should be concerned about eating too much fat overall, but not about eating prawns, brains, liver, and kidney, which, although high in cholesterol, are low in other fats. The important point is still to reduce the proportion of saturated fats in your diet.

- *Saturated fat* is found mainly in animal sources, such as red meat and dairy products. This type of fat can raise blood cholesterol.

- *Monounsaturated fat* is found in olive oil. This has no known effect on blood cholesterol and can be used in moderation.

- *Polyunsaturated fat* is found mainly in vegetable oils such as corn oil and sunflower oil, in polyunsaturated margarines, and in oily fish. This can lower blood cholesterol when taken as part of a low-fat diet. (But remember, polyunsaturated fats contain the same high number of calories as other fats, so it's wise to go easy on them.)

Some foods, such as eggs and offal (animal viscera and trimmings removed in butchering), are rich in dietary cholesterol. However, the intake of cholesterol in the diet has a smaller effect on blood cholesterol than foods high in saturated fats.

## SALT AND SUGAR

- Too much salt is linked to high blood pressure, which increases the risk of stroke and heart attacks and also exacerbates existing health problems you may have.

- Sugar is bad for your teeth—and your figure. It can also create an artificially high blood sugar level, which can drop to below your normal level, making you feel weak, hungry, and tired. Sweet treats made with sugar, such as cakes, pies, puddings, cookies, and ice cream, should be once-a-week treats only.

Salt and sugar are our worst enemies when they're hidden away in processed foods. Read the nutritional information labels on packaged foods and try to buy less of the ones that contain high added sugar and salt. (Note that many labels can be deceptive, listing several different *kinds* of sugar, sucrose, glucose, honey, corn syrup, and so on.) When cooking at home, try to use less salt during cooking (and preferably sea salt, which is lower in sodium than table salt), and none at the table (use flavor enhancers instead, or herbs, or lemon juice).

If you have trouble giving up, try buying a salt shaker with smaller holes. People tend to shake for the same amount of time, regardless of the amount of salt they're sprinkling on their food. Steam vegetables instead of boiling them. Steaming enhances their flavor and you won't miss the salt you add when you boil them. Use herbs and spices in casseroles as alternative flavorings.

Cut down on your sweet ingredients by making them part of a meal, and restrict them to once a day only. Alternative flavorings—dried fruit and "sweet" spices, like cinnamon, nutmeg, and cloves—can taste just as good in baking as sugar, and they're much better for you.

### THE IMPORTANCE OF A HIGH-FIBER DIET

For years dieters have been looking for a miracle substance that would help them lose weight. What they didn't know was that the very thing they desire has been literally right under their noses all along: the natural fiber in foods.

People in the developing world, have a lower incidence of heart disease, digestive illness, and obesity than Westerners. Why? Because their diets were rich in the natural fiber ours lacked.

By the early eighties most of us were locked into a pattern of buying and eating mostly processed foods from which the fiber had been "conveniently" removed by food processing plants: white bread, cornflakes, and white rice, for example. Our average intake of fiber was just less than 1 ounce a day, compared to a typical 2–5 ounces a day among people living in developing countries.

By boosting our fiber intake, by eating more wholemeal pasta and bread and whole-grain rice, potatoes with their skins on, legumes (such as lentils, beans, and peas), we can lose weight without feeling hungry.

As well as helping you to slim down, fiber in your diet takes good care of your digestive system, and keeps your bowels healthy. (Many older people take digestive fiber, such as Metamucil, regularly—ironically, to replace the very fiber that food processing has removed.)

The World Health Organization recommends that dietary fiber makes up at least 50 percent of our diet.

*Seven good reasons for eating fiber:*

1. A fat-rich diet passes relatively quickly through the stomach, but lingers in the bowel, where nutrients and water are extracted and the remaining waste material becomes small and difficult to propel, causing constipation and irregular bowel movements.

A high-fiber diet passes more slowly through the stomach, but speeds through the bowel, easing constipation and making bowel movements more regular and less of a strain.

2. High-fiber food stays longer in your stomach because it takes longer for the gastric acids to break it down. While your stomach remains full, your appetite is suppressed: a great boon for dieters!

3. Because it's such hard work for your gastric acids to break down the fibrous cell-wall material of high-fiber food, some of it will pass undigested to the bowel, which means you gain less weight because you don't absorb all the calories you consume.

4. Fiber also reduces your cravings for sweet and fatty foods, because it slows down and evens out the rate at which sugar is released into your blood, and also the rate at which it's cleared away.

The amount of sugar circulating in the blood is controlled by a hormone called insulin, and the amount of fiber in your diet is thought to have an effect on the amount of insulin you produce. After eating apples, apple puree, or apple juice, for example, your blood sugar level will rise. The fiber in the solid apple helps the blood sugar level to return to its normal level, whereas, after drinking filtered (clear) apple juice on its own, which contains no fiber, your blood sugar level will drop below normal.

5. A high-fiber diet is thought to help reduce the risk of bowel cancer because:

- ◆ A low-fiber diet results in small, hard stools with a higher concentration of whatever carcinogenic chemicals are present in the feces. The bulky stools of a high-fiber diet will have a lower concentration.

- ◆ The slow transit time of low-fiber feces through the bowel gives any carcinogens present more time in contact with the bowel walls, allowing it time to cause mischief with your system.

6. The risk of coronary heart disease is also thought to be reduced with a high-fiber diet. Certain soluble fiber (such

as oats, fruit, vegetables, and legumes) can help to lower blood cholesterol levels.

7. High-fiber foods contain healthy complex carbohydrates, which, as well as providing fiber, contain essential vitamins and minerals.

## THE IDEAL DIET

You may be surprised to learn that the ideal diet is the Mediterranean diet, which is less about losing weight and more about eating healthily, so that you can follow it even if you don't have to lose weight. Although you don't have to cut out red meat altogether, research shows that a diet of whole-grain bread, pasta, olive oil, fish, vegetables, fruit, garlic, fresh herbs, and red wine has a significant protective effect against heart disease.

- ◆ At least 50 percent of your daily energy should come from complex carbohydrates, such as whole-grain rice and pasta and legumes.

- ◆ You should eat 400 to 800 grams (about 14 oz. to 1½ lb.) of fresh fruit and raw or lightly steamed vegetables (not potatoes) a day.

- ◆ Eat more nuts (unsalted), seeds, legumes, and fish, which are rich in the essential fatty acids that help lower harmful blood cholesterol levels.

- ◆ Less than 30 percent of your daily energy should come from fat. Use more olive oil (which should be stored in cool dark conditions for it to offer the best benefits to your health) and less butter.

- Eat fish two or three times a week, try to have one or two vegetarian days every week, and try to eat red meat no more than once or twice a week.

*The best methods for preparing food include:*

- Eating fruit and vegetables raw or only lightly steamed (save the water for drinking or making a stock, as it contains some steamed-out nutrients).

- Grilling food with only a light brushing of olive or canola oil

- Baking

- Steaming

- Boiling with only minimal amounts of water and no added salt

- Poaching in vegetable stock

- Stir-frying using a light brushing of olive or canola oil

- Roasting only if the meat is on a rack so that the juice and fat run away

- Making low-fat gravies using granules and vegetable water (from steaming, above) instead of the meat juices

## Exercise

If you don't exercise regularly, you probably have a hundred and one excuses for not doing so. Being too busy is a common one. Another is that exercise will cause damage to your body, which is entirely untrue. Regular exercise is essential to keep our heart healthy and prevent heart disease. It also helps us cope with stress, looks after our lungs, and enables us to relax and even sleep better.

If we put our minds to it, most of us can find the time to do some form of exercise every day. It needn't mean "sport," or "athletics," as in running a marathon or doing aerobics. Brisk walking, swimming, and bicycling are all extremely beneficial forms of exercise. Some people working at high-pressure jobs even do exercises at their desks or using common office furniture. In fact, making these activities part of your routine can become such a pleasure that you'll feel lost and irritable when you're prevented from doing them.

Ideally, the exercise you choose should:

- Be pleasurable, to boost self-esteem, and to give you a little break from the rigors of your day

- Be carried out daily at the same time every day, so that your body will come to rely on this regular release of tension

- Last at least 20 minutes, uninterrupted, three times a week, to start off with, gradually increasing to half an hour or more five days a week

Regular exercise means:

- Your heart won't have to work as hard as when you aren't exercising.

- Your blood pressure will be lowered, because an exercised muscle needs less blood flow than an untrained one.

- Your glucose tolerance will improve (reducing the possibility of developing diabetes).

- The oxygen supply to your muscles will also improve.
- Your blood will be less likely to clot.
- Fat will be reduced and replaced by muscle.
- You'll lose excess weight.

If you're starting a new exercise routine and have previously been quite inactive, start slowly (for example, walk for ten minutes every day), and then build up to regular weekly times when you swim, bicycle, jog, or dance to keep fit.

## Smoking

According to the American Cancer Society, the best way to give up is to stop smoking by going cold turkey. That means, stopping abruptly *all* smoking at once. Other methods include nicotine fading (switching to lower tar and nicotine cigarettes), tapering (cutting down the number of cigarettes you smoke before quitting entirely), or setting a "quit date" (choosing a nonstressful time to quit while preparing yourself and your family and friends so that they can help you).

A nonprofit organization in Great Britain, QUIT, offers the following practical help to people who want to stop smoking.

1. Make a date to stop smoking completely—and stick to it.

2. Keep yourself busy to help you get through the first few days. Throw away all your ashtrays, unopened cigarette packs (including those you've hidden throughout the house), matches, and lighters.

3. Drink lots of water, and keep a glass by your side that you can sip steadily. (Carry a sports-jug of water on your commute to work.)

4. Be more active. This will help you relax. Join an exercise class, go for a walk, or have a swim.

5. Think positive. Withdrawal signs, although unpleasant, should be welcomed because they're positive signs that your body is recovering from the effects of tobacco. Common symptoms include headaches, sore throats, and irritability. They'll all disappear within a week or two.

6. Change your routine. If you bought your cigarettes on your usual route to work, go another way for a few days, or as long as you have to, in order to remove the temptation. If you smoked with friends after work at a bar, or out on the sidewalk during workday breaks, go somewhere else and do something different.

7. Don't make excuses. A crisis or a celebration is no excuse for "just one" cigarette. One leads to another, and another.

8. Treat yourself. Use the money you've saved on cigarettes for something special.

9. Watch what you eat. Eat fruit instead of fatty snacks if you're feeling jittery.

10. Take one day at a time, and remember: each day is good news for your health, your family, and your finances.

## Alcohol

If you drink more than 14 ounces of alcohol a week if you're a woman or 21 units if you're a man, you might find it helpful to keep a drink diary to monitor when, where, and with whom you drink the most. This will help you work out ways of cutting down.

- Try to keep one or two days a week alcohol-free.

- Sip drinks slowly and stick to smaller measures. Don't feel obliged to keep up with other drinkers. And alternate alcoholic drinks with mineral water or juice, to reduce your total alcoholic intake.

- If you're finding it hard to cut down, confidential advice and guidance are available from a number of organizations, including Alcoholics Anonymous, Al-Anon, and Alateen. Many HMOs (health maintenance organizations) offer support classes to help members reduce or stop their drinking (or their smoking).

## *Relaxing*

"Type A" people cope badly with stress and are *four times* more likely than the average person of their age group to develop coronary heart disease.

Type A people:

- Are competitive, aggressive, and impatient
- Are angry and easily irritated
- Are frenzied and constantly trying to meet self-imposed deadlines
- Lack self-esteem
- Swear a lot and are critical of others
- Can't sit still and do nothing
- Generate guilt and a sense of failure in others

If you have any five or six of these traits, you are a type A.

Type B people:

- Have no time urgency
- Have no free-floating hostility
- Have no desire to take control
- Are satisfied with their self-esteem
- Rarely swear
- Are understanding and compassionate

Here are some ways to modify type A behavior and reduce stress:

- Make an effort to be more flexible.
- Try to be more affectionate, and take time to listen to others.
- Practice meditation and deep-breathing exercises, which slow down your usual frenzied pace.
- When you're under stress, ask yourself whether what's bothering you now will matter tomorrow, next week, next month, or next year. Learn to put your life in perspective.
- Use counseling to learn to better cope with life's major problems.

Better "mood-management" skills will also help you cope with the usual build up of trivial irritations.

Instead of bottling up anger, let it out—but not on other people. We usually take out our anger toward our families on people at work, and our anger toward our colleagues on our families (or our pets). Instead, try some of the following:

- Shut yourself in your own room or even retreat under your "comforter" (a well-named item of bedroom linen!), imagine the person who has made you angry, and shout at them out loud. You'll feel much better for it, and so will your family.

- Keep a diary. Writing down your thoughts can reduce your feelings of conflict anger.

- Make some time for yourself every day, time in which you do something you want, but don't need, to do.

- Find a simple phrase you can repeat to yourself (perhaps while doing deep-breathing exercises), such as "I can handle this," "I'm doing well," "I sense that I'm calmer," or "I feel good."

## *Water*

Although garlic has definite health benefits, it can, like so many other substances in our diet and lifestyle, place a demand on the body, according to the naturopathic nutritionist Barbara Wren. Vitamin supplements have the same effect, and Wren says that you'll get the best benefit from garlic by ensuring that your body isn't dehydrated. If it is, it'll be unable to make good use of the vitamins and minerals in the garlic.

To determine if you need to drink more water, ask yourself the following questions:

1. *Do you suffer from any of the following symptoms?*

- Fatigue
- Constipation
- Insomnia or lack of sleep

- Indigestion
- PMS and/or mood swings
- Lack of energy
- Allergies
- Infertility
- Fluid retention

These are the most common reasons people turn to supplements, but they're also signs that we should be removing toxins from our body instead of putting in more stuff—whether healthful supplements *or* drugs.

2. *Are you dehydrated?*

Do you:

- Suffer from stress?
- Drink large volumes of tea, coffee, or alcohol?
- Eat a lot of junk food?
- Travel a good deal, especially by air?
- Work in an air-conditioned office?
- Use a computer monitor or other video display terminal?
- Smoke?
- Take any drugs?

Barbara Wren says:

Most of us do a lot of these things, and then suffer with various symptoms and decide to take a supplement—which just adds to the stress and dehydration we're already under. The body responds by protecting the cell membranes with a shell of cholesterol to keep all the fluids intact inside each cell. But if these fluids are trapped inside the cells too long they become stagnant and toxic, causing more health problems.

3. *Could you drink more water, and improve your diet?*
To rehydrate, we should all aim to drink 8 large glasses (2 quarts) of plain water every day. (Don't include the water contained in fruit juice in this goal.) This helps the body get rid of trapped toxins, and restores normal levels of energy and good health.

Adding more rice, fresh vegetables, and legumes to your diet helps with the rehydration process as well as providing the balance of minerals and vitamins your body needs.

Once your body has gotten used to your drinking more water and eating more rice, vegetables, and legumes, you may need to add essential fatty acids, such as evening primrose oil or linseeds, and an emulsifier such as lecithin (ask at your favorite health food store), which allows the body to use the oils it needs. Together, these can combat problems like lethargy, but they won't not work unless you first go through the detoxification process described above.

## Changing to a Healthier Lifestyle

### ANN'S STORY

Ann has always known that she is at high risk of developing heart disease. Her mother died of heart failure when

Ann was just 7, and her father died of a heart attack when Ann was 27. "On top of that, I'd had rheumatic fever as a child, and this is a condition that increases the risk of heart disease," Ann says.

> I was aware of how to live a healthy life, not smoking, drinking little or no alcohol, and cutting down on fatty foods. But I had a weight problem that I just couldn't fix, and this terrified me, because excess weight is yet another risk for heart disease (as well as causing other health and mobility complications).
>
> Then I read about Kwai garlic supplements, which were being promoted as part of the Mediterranean diet as a way of getting fitter and losing weight. As I read the article, I thought of my lovely little grandchildren, and I realized that this might be my only hope if I wanted to live long enough to see them grow up.
>
> I started the diet, and despite having failed at every other diet I've ever tried I lost 22 pounds over the next 12 months. I wasn't even aware that I was dieting or losing weight, for I never felt hungry. The diet differed from others I'd tried in that I had to increase the amount of fruit and oily fish I ate. But the only other difference was the fact that I was taking a garlic supplement, so I can only assume this contributed to my weight loss. I eat garlic anyway, with my food. But this was the first time I'd taken it as a supplement.
>
> When I had a cold or a touch of hay fever I upped my dose slightly—because you can't overdose on garlic—and my symptoms disappeared almost immediately.

I now take two Kwai tablets a day, and my diet is as follows: cereal or scrambled eggs and toast for breakfast, fish with salad for lunch, and a light supper of salad, dressed with olive oil and lemon juice, or a home-made vegetable soup. I have snacks of fruit during the day, and a variety of fruit for dessert too. I also drink a lot of water, and I feel just great, as if I could take on the world.

But I know it's not all in my mind. When my blood was recently tested, my LDL levels were low, and my HDL was high—the perfect healthy balance.

## Using Garlic

Now we come to the point you've been waiting for—about how to *use* garlic in the real world in which you have to mingle with other people. Do you eat it raw or cooked? Are garlic supplements better or worse than fresh garlic, or more effective, or more offputting with others you face every day? And if you *do* take supplements, should you choose pearles or tablets? There's some debate about this.

The first school of thought says that it's the allicin in garlic that's its principal active component. This is the substance that causes a raw clove of garlic or an onion to smell when it's cut open. Allicin starts to degrade from the moment it's produced, and particularly rapidly if it's heated. Therefore, if garlic is heated in any way, its main benefits are destroyed. This argument goes on to say that only raw or powdered garlic is any good if you want to reduce your cholesterol levels. This means that cooked garlic, including garlic oil (which is processed by steaming garlic), is ineffective.

However, a team led by Dr. Philip Barlow, at the University of Humberside, Great Britain, looked into the claims that dried garlic is the best source of allicin when compared with garlic oil, and found that few of the products tested (dried garlic powder and garlic oil used in capsules) contained *any* allicin at all. Therefore, they say, the activity of garlic as a means of lowering the cholesterol in the blood is linked to the sulfides that derive from the allicin as it breaks down and takes up oxygen from the surrounding air.

Dr. Reg Saynor, author of *The Garlic Effect* (Hodder & Stoughton), researched the effects of onions (also in the allium family, with garlic) on the blood fats of patients with heart disease, and found that the benefits were the same whether the onion was raw, boiled, or fried. He claims that the same apparently holds true for garlic, and this strongly suggests that allicin, which is destroyed by heating, is not in itself responsible for garlic's health benefits.

Fresh garlic varies enormously in quality and strength, the strongest supposedly being Chinese garlic, which is often commercially available in Asian markets in certain cities in the United States and which is used to make Kwai garlic tablets. A 300-mg. daily dose of Kwai is the equivalent of half a clove of Chinese garlic. Because of the wide variation in fresh garlic, Professor Edzard Ernst recommends 4 grams daily, that is, half to one clove of fresh garlic (of the ordinary kind available in your supermarket.

Weighing the research available, I advise the following:

- Try to include *both* raw and cooked garlic in your diet. Make it an everyday seasoning. People in the garlic-eating Mediterranean countries (where heart disease is lower than in non garlic-eating countries) cook their garlic just as often as they eat it raw.

## Tips for Using Garlic

- A study comparing garlic oil capsules with garlic powder tablets showed that people preferred to take tablets because they generally felt healthier.

- If you find it difficult to tolerate raw garlic, try mixing it with fennel, dill or caraway, or take garlic powder tablets instead.

- Garlic products should not be given to children under six years old, but garlic can be safely added to their diet.

- Take your garlic supplements with meals to reduce the risk of developing an odor.

- As you add more garlic to your diet, the smell will become less noticeable.

- Appearances can be deceptive: smaller cloves of garlic often produce the most flavor.

- Taking garlic tablets with a fatty meal will help your body absorb much less fat from the food.

- Instead of crushing garlic in a metal press, which can add a crude flavor to the garlic, squash it under a knife. Add salt to stop it from dispersing over the chopping board, but don't add additional salt to your cooking.

- Use a supplement that suits you if you don't like the taste of fresh garlic, or you have a specific problem like a high cholesterol level or high blood pressure that you want to address. But involve your doctor in your plans.

- Consult with your doctor if you have a health problem, such as a bleeding disorder, and have been advised not to use aspirin. Garlic may have a similar effect in thinning the blood, and although this is beneficial to most of us, there are suggestions that for some people garlic may be potentially hazardous.

*Five tips for coping with garlic breath:*

1. Chew a little fresh parsley or mint (some people grow them in a window box, for use also with foods or teas), or the bitter herb rue.

2. Try swallowing a whole clove of garlic. You'll smell as sweet as anyone who takes no garlic.

3. Follow the French, and have a glass of red wine.

4. Suck a slice of lemon.

5. If you're taking garlic medicinally, mince it and add it to something you can swallow without chewing. Joan and Lydia Wilen, authors of *Garlic—Nature's Super Healer*, recommend using a spoonful of fat-free yogurt, which acts as a buffer for the garlic.

# 5

# Garlic Recipes

*Note:* Measures are given in both metric (which some cooks prefer) and U.S. equivalents (the conversions are approximate, having been rounded up or down). Use either system—not a mixture of the two—in any recipe. All spoon measures are level unless stated otherwise.

# Soups & Salads

## Avocado Soup

*Serves 4*

2 ripe avocados
500 g./18 oz. carton cottage cheese or other skimmed-
    milk soft cheese
900 ml./1½ pints tomato juice
1 clove garlic, crushed

Peel, pit, and chop the avocados. Put them (in two or three batches) in a blender or food processor with the cheese, tomato juice, and garlic and work to a smooth soup.

Chill for 2 hours before serving.

## Chilled Almond and Garlic Soup

*Serves 4*

This is meant to be a thick soup, but if necessary you can thin it with a little extra milk.

> 1 large head garlic
> 1 large Spanish onion, roughly chopped
> 900 ml./1½ pints milk
> 125 g./4 oz. ground almonds
> juice of 1 small lemon
> 2 teaspoons paprika
> 3–4 pinches cayenne pepper
> salt

Separate and peel the garlic cloves. Put them in a fairly large saucepan with the chopped onion and add 300 ml./½ pint of the milk. Bring to a boil, cover the pan, and then simmer very gently for 20–25 minutes, until the onions and garlic are very soft.

Pour into a food processor, add the ground almonds, and whiz into a smooth paste.

Tip the paste into the saucepan and stir in the remaining 600 ml./1 pint milk. Season generously with salt. Bring the soup to a boil, stirring all the while, and then simmer, still stirring, for 8–10 minutes. Pour into a bowl and let stand to cool. Then chill in the refrigerator.

Before serving, mix the lemon juice with the paprika and cayenne pepper in a cup, using a teaspoon. Pour the chilled soup into individual bowls and spoon a whirl of the lemon, paprika, and cayenne mixture on top of each bowl.

# Garlic Soup

*Serves 4*

16 large cloves garlic, unpeeled
1 teaspoon salt
a dash of black pepper
1 teaspoon mixed dried herbs
2 cloves
4 sprigs parsley
3 egg yolks
3 tablespoons olive oil

Bring the garlic to a boil in 900 ml./1½ pints of water in a covered pan with the salt, pepper, herbs, cloves, and parsley. Then simmer briskly for 30 minutes.

Meanwhile, beat the egg yolks in a bowl and stir in the olive oil, drop by drop, to make a thick mayonnaise base.

Beat a little of the hot garlic liquid into the egg mixture. Then, very gradually, strain in the rest through a sieve (pressing the juice out of the garlic cloves with a spoon), stirring the soup vigorously all the while. Serve immediately.

## Gazpacho

*Serves 4*

- 450 g./1 lb. tomatoes, peeled
- 1 diced cucumber, peeled
- 2 cloves garlic, chopped
- 1 spring onion, finely sliced
- 12 black olives, pitted
- a few strips green pepper
- 3 tablespoons olive oil
- 1 tablespoon wine vinegar
- salt and pepper
- 1 pinch cayenne pepper
- a sprinkle of fresh marjoram, mint, or parsley, chopped
- 300 ml./½ pint iced water
- 4 cubes ice, roughly crushed
- a few cubes coarse brown bread to garnish

Chop the tomatoes until almost pureed. Stir in all the other ingredients. Keep very cold until it's time to serve the soup, and then thin with the iced water, garnish with the bread, and serve with broken-up ice floating in the bowl. A couple of hard-boiled eggs, coarsely chopped, also make a good addition.

## Vegetable Soup with Garlic and Tomato Sauce

*Serves 6–8*

500 g./1 lb. green beans, cut into 5 cm./2 inch lengths
500 g./1 lb. fresh pinto beans or fava beans, shelled
500 g./1 lb. fresh white haricot beans, shelled, or 250 g./8 oz. dried haricot or cannellini beans (large white beans), soaked overnight
2 medium potatoes, peeled and roughly chopped
2 tomatoes, peeled
500 g./1 lb. zucchini (unpeeled), diced
whites of two leeks, chopped
leaves of two celery sticks, chopped
salt and pepper
100 g./4 oz. large short macaroni

**PISTOU SAUCE**
3–4 garlic cloves, peeled
2 large bunches fresh basil
100 g./4 oz. grated gruyere or Parmesan cheese
1 tomato, grilled, with skin and seeds removed
2–3 tablespoons olive oil

Bring 2 liters/3½ pints of cold water to a boil, and add all the vegetables except the green beans and zucchini. Season with salt and pepper. Cover and simmer gently for 2 hours. Add the remaining vegetables and the macaroni, adding more salt and pepper if necessary, and cook for another 15 minutes. (Alternatively, you can precook the dried beans, simmer the fresh vegetables until tender, and add the cooked beans to the soup at the same time as the macaroni.)

In the meantime, make the pistou sauce. Pound the garlic and basil together into a paste with a pestle and mortar, and then work in the cheese and the grilled tomato. Add the olive oil, a little at a time, beating in well, and then add a few spoonfuls of the soup broth.

Serve the sauce in its mortar with the soup, warm or hot.

## Cacik—Greek Yogurt and Cucumber Salad

*Serves 4*

> 2 tablespoons olive oil
> 1 teaspoon wine vinegar
> 1 clove garlic, crushed
> 175 g./6 oz. natural yogurt
> 5 cm./2 inch piece of cucumber, peeled and diced finely
>     or grated coarsely
> 3–4 fresh mint leaves, chopped finely, or
>     ½ teaspoon dried mint
> salt

Lightly beat the oil, vinegar, and garlic with a fork in a bowl. Add the yogurt and beat until smooth and well amalgamated. Add the cucumber, salt, and chopped mint and mix thoroughly. Serve chilled.

## Chicken Avocado Salad

*Serves 4*

1.2 kg./2½ lb. free-range roasting chicken
2 teaspoons curry powder
1 carrot, split lengthwise
1 stick celery, chopped roughly
1 onion, halved
1 bouquet garni
1 bay leaf
1 teaspoon black peppercorns
50 g./2 oz. dried apricots
150 ml./¼ pint orange juice
2 ripe avocados
50 g./2 oz. sunflower seeds

DRESSING
90 ml./3 oz. natural yogurt
¼ teaspoon curry powder
1 clove garlic, crushed

Rub the chicken with the curry powder. Put it in a saucepan with the carrot, celery, onion, bouquet garni, bay leaf, and peppercorns. Pour in enough water to just cover the legs. Bring to a boil, cover, and simmer for 50 minutes, or until the chicken is tender. Lift out the chicken and leave until completely cool (for at least 4 hours, or overnight in the refrigerator).

Soak the apricots in the orange juice for at least 4 hours. Cut all the chicken meat from the bones and dice it. Peel, pit, and dice 1½ avocados. Cut the remaining ½ avocado into thin strips. Drain and finely chop the apricots.

In a bowl, mix together the chicken, diced avocado, apricots, and sunflower seeds. Beat together the yogurt, curry powder, and garlic. Fold the resulting dressing into the salad.

Place the salad on a serving plate and garnish with the reserved strips of avocado. Serve immediately.

## Mushroom Salad with Garlic and Green Pepper Sauce

*Serves 2–3*

> 175 g./6 oz. button mushrooms, sliced
> 3 tablespoons vegetable oil
>
> SAUCE
> 2 green peppers
> 2 large cloves garlic, unpeeled
> 2 tablespoons fresh fennel leaves, chopped
> 1 tablespoon olive oil

Heat the oil in a frying pan and saute the mushrooms very quickly. Drain and cool. Boil the peppers and garlic together for 6 minutes, and then drain. Pop the garlic out of its skin (or smash with the flat of a knife and remove skin). Blend the peppers and garlic with the fennel and the olive oil. Spoon the sauce over the mushrooms. Chill.

## Salad Niçoise

*Serves 6*

50 g./2 oz. can anchovy fillets or one 250 g./8 oz. can tuna fish
4 eggs, hard-boiled
1 cucumber
1 large green pepper
1 red pepper
6 spring onions
6 large tomatoes
1 garlic clove
225 g./8 oz. very young fava beans, podded (in season)
100 g./4 oz. small Nice olives
1 teaspoon lemon juice
4 basil leaves, torn into small pieces
4 tablespoons virgin olive oil
salt and pepper

Chop up the anchovy fillets, or shred the tuna fish with a fork. Slice the hard-boiled eggs. Peel and thinly slice the cucumber. Slice the peppers, discarding the seeds, and slice the spring onions and tomatoes. Peel and halve the garlic clove.

Rub the sides of a large salad bowl well with the cut garlic. Layer the anchovy or tuna, eggs, and vegetable ingredients alternately in the bowl with the fava beans and olives. Season with plenty of pepper and a little salt.

Prepare a vinaigrette with the lemon juice, torn basil leaves, and olive oil and pour over the salad. Toss lightly and serve chilled.

## Tuna, Bean, and Potato Salad

*Serves 4*

350 g./12 oz. new potatoes
198 g./7 oz. can tuna fish, drained and flaked
432 g./15½ oz. can borlotti beans, drained
2 shallots or small onions, thinly sliced
shredded lettuce

DRESSING
1 clove garlic
1 teaspoon Dijon mustard
2 tablespoons wine vinegar
4 tablespoons olive oil
1 tablespoon chopped parsley
salt and pepper

Cook the potatoes in boiling salted water for about 20 minutes, until tender. Drain and leave to cool. Cut into quarters if they're large and place in a bowl.

Gently stir in the tuna, beans, and shallots or onions.

Place the dressing ingredients in a screw-top jar and shake well to mix. Pour over the salad and mix lightly.

Serve on shredded lettuce with warm whole grain bread.

# VEGETABLES

# Baked Eggplant

*Serves 6*

> 6 large eggplant
> salt and pepper
> 10 tomatoes
> olive oil
> 6 tablespoons fine breadcrumbs
> 225 g./8 oz. fresh parsley, finely chopped
> 6 basil leaves, chopped
> 4 cloves garlic

Slice the eggplant without peeling them. Sprinkle with salt, cover with a clean kitchen towel, and leave to sweat for 1 hour.

Preheat the oven to 425°F.

Peel, seed, and slice the tomatoes. Rinse the eggplant slices and pat them dry with a cloth.

Grease a baking dish with plenty of olive oil. Line with a layer of eggplant, and then a layer of the sliced tomatoes. Cover with a good quantity of persillade, made by mixing together the breadcrumbs, parsley, basil, and crushed garlic. Season with salt and pepper and repeat with a second (and maybe even a third) layer of vegetables, finishing with a layer of the persillade. Drizzle a tablespoon of olive oil over the dish.

Bake in the preheated oven for 35–40 minutes. Leave to cool overnight. Serve cold.

## Carrots with Garlic and Ginger

*Serves 3–4*

> 1 tablespoon cumin seeds
> 450 g./1 lb. young carrots, sliced
> 1 large clove garlic, crushed
> 2.5 cm./1 inch piece root ginger, peeled and grated
> 2 tablespoons soy sauce

Preheat the oven to 375°F. Put the cumin seeds on a baking tray and cook for 5 minutes, until lightly toasted, shaking them around from time to time. Put to one side.

Steam the carrots in a colander or steamer over simmering water until they're cooked but still crunchy.

Mix the garlic and ginger into the soy sauce and toss the carrots in it, mixing well. Sprinkle with the cumin seeds just before serving.

## Garlic Mushrooms

*Serves 4*

450 g./1 lb. mushrooms
175 g./6 oz. butter, at room temperature
2 cloves garlic, crushed
1 tablespoon lemon juice
1–2 tablespoons freshly chopped parsley
salt and freshly ground black pepper

Preheat the oven to 425°F.

Prepare the mushrooms by simply wiping them with kitchen paper, and then pull off the stalks—but don't discard them.

In a small bowl, combine the crushed garlic with the butter, and stir in the parsley and lemon juice. Season the mixture with salt and freshly ground black pepper.

Arrange the mushroom caps, upside down, in a gratin dish or roasting pan, with the stalks among them. Put a little of the garlic butter mixture in each cap, spreading whatever remains over the stalks.

Place the dish on the top rack of the preheated oven and cook for 10–15 minutes, or until the butter is sizzling away and the mushrooms look slightly toasted. Serve straight from the oven with slices of crusty bread to mop up the garlicky juices.

## Garlic Potatoes

*Serves 6*

> 1 kg./2 lb. waxy potatoes
> 110 ml./4 oz. olive oil
> 2 cloves garlic, crushed
> 2 tablespoons finely chopped parsley
> sea salt and black pepper

Peel and wash the potatoes. Dry them well and cut into regular slices about ¼ inch thick.

Heat the oil in a large frying pan. Add the potatoes. Mix well so that each potato is coated in oil. Add the crushed garlic and parsley, mix well, and cover the pan. Lower the heat and cook gently, turning the potatoes every 5 minutes until golden brown on all sides. Replace the lid each time. Cook until tender.

Season with freshly ground sea salt and black pepper and serve.

# Pumpkin and Garlic Gratin

This dish is excellent either on its own with a crisp winter salad or as an accompaniment to a simple roast.

*Serves 6*

- 1 kg./2 lb. pumpkin, peeled and chopped into small cubes
- ½ cup rice, boiled for 10 minutes and drained well
- 1 handful grated gruyere cheese
- 4 tablespoons flour, sieved
- 3 cloves garlic, finely chopped
- 5 tablespoons fresh thyme, finely chopped
- ½ teaspoon freshly grated nutmeg
- salt and pepper
- 100 g./4 oz. breadcrumbs (optional)
- olive oil

Preheat the oven to 325°F.

Toss together all the ingredients except the breadcrumbs until the pumpkin is well covered with flour and herbs. Put into a well-oiled gratin dish and cover with breadcrumbs. Drizzle with olive oil and bake until the top is crusty and a deep caramel brown. The pumpkin will have an almost purée-like consistency.

# Ratatouille

*Serves 6–8*

> 450 g./1 lb. eggplant, cut into 10 mm./½ inch slices
> salt and pepper
> olive oil
> 450 g./1 lb. zucchini, cut into small chunks
> 450 g./1 lb. mixed red and green peppers, cored and thinly sliced
> 225 g./8 oz. onions, peeled and finely chopped
> 700 g./1½ lb. tomatoes, peeled, seeded, and chopped
> 3 cloves garlic, peeled and finely chopped
> ½ teaspoon sugar
> a handful of parsley, finely chopped
> leaves from several sprigs of thyme
> 9–10 basil leaves, cut into strips

Sprinkle the eggplants with salt and set to drain for 30 minutes. Pat dry and cut into small chunks. Heat about 6 tablespoons of olive oil in a large, heavy-based frying pan. Add the eggplant and when brown on all sides, remove and drain on paper towels.

Add a little more oil to the pan and fry the zucchini until all their moisture has evaporated. Remove and drain. Continue with the peppers, removing them when tender.

Then cook the onions, until soft but not brown. Stir in the tomatoes, garlic, sugar, parsley, and thyme and simmer for about 30 minutes. Add the rest of the vegetables. After 5 minutes, remove from the heat, mix in the basil, and refrigerate overnight.

Serve cold or reheat.

## Stir-fried Peppers and Water Chestnuts

*Serves 4*

- 2 green peppers
- 1 red pepper
- 230 g./8 oz. can water chestnuts
- 6 spring onions
- 25 g./1 oz. root ginger, grated or finely chopped
- 4 tablespoons groundnut or sunflower oil
- 1 clove garlic, finely chopped
- 125 g./4 oz. beansprouts
- 4 tablespoons dry sherry or stock
- 2 tablespoons soy sauce

Core and deseed the peppers and cut them into ¾ inch squares.

Drain and thinly slice the water chestnuts.

Cut the spring onions into ¾ inch lengths.

Peel and finely grate the root ginger.

Heat the oil in a wok or large frying pan on high heat. Put in the peppers, water chestnuts, spring onions, ginger, and garlic and stir-fry for 2 minutes. Add the beansprouts and stir-fry for 1 minute more. Add the sherry or stock and soy sauce and stir-fry for a further 30 seconds.

Serve at once. Basmati rice makes a good accompaniment.

## Golden Raisin and Peanut Pilaf

*Serves 4*

> 3 tablespoons sunflower oil
> 1 medium onion, thinly sliced
> 1 clove garlic, chopped
> 1 teaspoon ground coriander
> 1 teaspoon cumin seeds
> 250 g./8 oz. long-grain brown rice
> 600 ml./1 pint vegetable stock
> 1 pinch sea salt
> 40 g./1½ oz. unsalted peanuts, shelled
> 40 g./1½ oz. golden raisins

Heat the oil in a saucepan on a low heat. Add the onion and garlic and cook for 2 minutes. Mix in the coriander and cumin and continue cooking until the onion is soft. Add the rice and stir for 1 minute.

Pour in the stock, add the salt, and bring to a boil. Cover the pan, and cook over low heat until the rice is tender and all the stock has been absorbed.

Turn off the heat, but leave the pan on the burner. Stir the peanuts and raisins into the rice. Replace the lid and let the rice stand for another 10 minutes before serving.

# CHEESE, SAUCES, DIPS & NUTS

## Garlic Cheese

*Serves 6*

> 450 g./1 lb. cream cheese
> ½ garlic clove, crushed
> salt and pepper
> a dash of red wine vinegar

Mix all the ingredients together with a fork, and then transfer to a deep earthenware dish. Keep refrigerated. Eat with crusty bread.

## Garlic Cheese Flan

*Serves 4–6*

PASTRY CASE
125 g./4 oz. butter or margarine
175 g./6 oz. plain flour
4 tablespoons cold water
salt

FILLING
450 g./1 lb. fresh broccoli florets
100 g./4 oz. mushrooms, sliced
1 small bunch parsley, finely chopped
1 large clove garlic, finely chopped
25 g./1 oz. sunflower margarine
100 g./4 oz. cheddar cheese, grated
2 free-range eggs
210 ml./7 oz. light cream
salt and pepper

Preheat the oven to 350°F.

To make the pastry, rub the butter or margarine into the flour and add a pinch of salt. Mix in the water and work to a smooth dough. Chill for 2 hours before rolling out.

Use the pastry to line a 10 inch flan dish. Lay the pastry over the dish with a rolling-pin, press into the edges, and roll off the surplus pastry. Cover the base with foil, weight with dry beans, and bake by itself for 10 minutes. Remove from the oven and cool.

Turn the oven down to 325°F.

Steam the broccoli florets in a colander or steamer over simmering water for about 5 minutes, until cooked through but still crisp. Arrange them over the base of the pastry case.

Heat the margarine in a frying pan and quickly fry the sliced mushrooms. Stir in the parsley and garlic, and season with salt and pepper. Spread this mixture over the broccoli and cover with the grated cheese.

Beat the eggs thoroughly and stir in the cream. Season with salt and pepper, pour over the flan, and bake for 45 minutes, or until set. Serve warm or cold.

## Aioli (Garlic Mayonnaise)

*Serves 6*

To prepare this classic garlic mayonnaise of Provence, make sure that all the ingredients are kept at room temperature for an hour beforehand.

- 10 garlic cloves
- a little salt
- ¼ teaspoon finely ground black pepper
- 2 free-range egg yolks
- 250 ml./8 oz. olive oil
- juice of 1 lemon
- 2 tablespoons lukewarm water

Peel the garlic cloves. Chop them coarsely and pound them in a mortar with the salt and pepper. Work in the egg yolks.

Add the olive oil drop by drop, stirring all the while. When half the oil has been added, stir in the lemon juice and water. Gradually add the rest of the oil. The finished product should be firmer than ordinary mayonnaise.

# Eggplant Pâté

*Serves 6*

750 g./½ lb. eggplant
2 cloves garlic, sliced
juice of half a lemon (or more, to taste)
5 tablespoons olive oil or good vegetable oil
salt and black pepper
black olives to garnish

Preheat the oven to 350°F.

Wash and dry the eggplant, prick them with a fork (otherwise they may explode in the oven), and cook them in the oven for one hour, turning them occasionally.

When the eggplant are cool enough to handle, halve them, scoop out their flesh into a sieve, and press lightly to extract their bitter juices. Put the flesh, with the garlic and lemon juice, into a blender or food processor and blend, adding the oil slowly at the same time, until quite smooth. Taste and adjust the seasoning.

Spread the pâté on a shallow platter and garnish with the olives. Serve with crusty baguettes or wholemeal crackers.

## Garlic Butter

This is lovely spread on French bread or rolls.

1 clove garlic
225 g./8 oz. butter
2 tablespoons parsley, chopped

Mash the garlic into the butter along with the parsley. Place in an insulated butter dish and chill well.

## Garlic-and-Bread Sauce

This sauce is served with vegetables or fish, either separately in bowls or poured over the dish.

*Serves 4–6*

> 3 medium-sized slices of crustless white bread, soaked in water for 10 minutes
> 2–3 cloves garlic, chopped
> 1 tablespoon white wine vinegar
> 4 tablespoons olive oil
> 50 g./2 oz. ground walnuts or ground almonds (optional)
> salt

Gently squeeze the bread, leaving it still quite moist. Place it in a blender or food processor with the chopped garlic, vinegar, and a little salt and blend until smooth.

Then slowly add the olive oil, while the blades are in motion. Add the ground nuts (if used) at the end and blend briefly.

The sauce should be of a runny consistency.

# Garlic Dip

*Serves 4*

    75 g./3 oz. cottage cheese
    1 tablespoon natural low-fat yogurt
    1 tablespoon thick Greek yogurt
    25 g./1 oz. dry-roasted peanuts
    1 clove garlic, crushed
    salt and pepper

Blend all the ingredients together, season to taste with salt and pepper, and chill.

Serve in a bowl in the center of a platter surrounded by thin sticks of carrot, cucumber, celery, and apple (cut the apple into a bowl of water with lemon juice, to prevent browning).

# Guacamole

*Serves 4 as a dip*

> 2 large ripe avocados
> 2 medium-sized tomatoes
> the juice of half a lemon
> 1 clove garlic, crushed
> 1 small bunch fresh cilantro leaves
> a splash of Tabasco sauce (according to taste)
> salt and pepper

Combine all the ingredients in a blender or food processor until smooth and creamy.

Turn into a serving dish and place the avocado pit in the center to prevent the mixture from turning brown.

Serve immediately.

## Humus

*Serves 4–6*

175 g./6 oz. chickpeas, picked clean and soaked overnight
2 cloves garlic, chopped
2 tablespoons tahini paste (optional, but add more oil if not used)
juice of 1½ lemons
1½ teaspoons ground cumin
4 tablespoons vegetable oil
300 ml./½ pint chickpea cooking liquid
salt and pepper

GARNISH
1–2 tablespoons olive oil or vegetable oil
a little cayenne pepper or paprika

Rinse the chickpeas. Cover with plenty of water in a large pan, bring to a boil, and skim until clear. Cover and cook until soft. In a pressure cooker they'll take 15–20 minutes, otherwise a little over an hour, according to their age. Strain the chickpeas, reserving the cooking liquid.

Divide the chickpeas and the remaining ingredients in two, and place the first batch in a blender or food processor. Blend until grainy and of a runny consistency. If too dry, add more liquid and then adjust the seasoning and blend it in briefly. Make the second batch in the same fashion.

Pour the humus onto a flat platter and sprinkle the oil and the cayenne pepper or paprika decoratively on top before serving.

## Sweet-Pepper Purée

*Serves 3–4*

> 3 large bell peppers, halved and deseeded (can be green, red, or yellow, or 1 of each for color)
> 4 cloves garlic, peeled
> juice of half a lemon
> 50 g./2 oz. sunflower margarine
> salt and pepper

Put the pepper halves into a pan with the whole cloves of garlic and cover with cold water. Bring to a boil, simmer for 10 minutes, and then drain. Blend with the lemon juice and margarine, and season to taste. Serve hot or cold.

## Sweet and Sour Peanuts

*Serves 4*

    half a small pineapple
    1 green pepper, deseeded and halved
    1 tablespoon cornflour
    2 teaspoons soy sauce
    5 tablespoons cider vinegar
    1 tablespoon clear honey
    3 tablespoons sunflower oil
    1 large onion, thinly sliced
    1 clove garlic, finely chopped
    125 g./4 oz. unsalted peanuts, shelled
    225 g./8 oz. can bamboo shoots, drained and thinly sliced
    225 g./8 oz. can water chestnuts, drained and thinly sliced

Cut the skin from the pineapple. Slice the flesh and cut into ¾ inch dice, removing the cores.

Cut the pepper into ¾ inch squares.

Put the cornflour in a bowl and gradually mix in the soy sauce, vinegar, and honey.

Heat the oil in a wok or large frying pan over a low heat. Add the pepper, onion, and garlic and stir-fry for 2 minutes. Put in the peanuts, bamboo shoots, and water chestnuts and stir-fry for another 2 minutes. Mix in the diced pineapple.

Stir the cornflour mixture and pour it into the pan. Simmer, stirring, until the mixture thickens to a glossy sauce. Remove from the heat and serve as soon as possible.

# PASTA

## Chickpea and Sausage Pasta

*Serves 6*

> 450 g./1 lb. chickpeas, soaked overnight in water with 1 teaspoon baking soda

4 leeks

1 carrot

5–6 spinach leaves (optional, but they do help soften the peas)

2 cloves garlic

1 bay leaf

5 sage leaves

1 large lean sausage or 6 small ones

¼ teaspoon grated nutmeg

salt and pepper

2 tablespoons fresh parsley, finely chopped, to garnish

75 g./3 oz. fresh pasta

grated gruyere (optional)

DRESSING
aioli (see page 105)

Soak the peas and rinse them well. Put them in a large saucepan with 6 pints of cold water, two leeks, and the carrot (all cut into easily retrievable pieces), the spinach leaves, garlic, bay leaf, and sage. Bring slowly to a boil, skim off any foam, cover tightly, and simmer gently for 2–3 hours until the peas are tender.

About half an hour before they're fully cooked, add the sausage to the chickpeas. When the chickpeas and sausage are done cooking remove them both from the broth.

Remove the cooked vegetables from the chickpeas, and then mix the peas with the aioli, one raw leek (sliced), and the nutmeg. Add salt and pepper to taste. Garnish with chopped parsley.

Strain the broth, slice the sausage, and add it to the broth with the remaining leek (finely sliced), the pasta, and salt and pepper. Cook until the pasta is just tender. Sprinkle with grated gruyere (if desired) before serving.

## Garlic and Broccoli Spaghetti

*Serves 4–5*

450 g./1 lb. sprouting broccoli
300 g./10 oz. spaghetti, uncooked
7 tablespoons virgin olive oil
2–3 cloves garlic, finely chopped
sea salt and black pepper
freshly grated Parmesan cheese (optional)

Wash the broccoli and cut into ½ inch pieces, discarding any hard, thick stalks. Put a little salted water in a saucepan and bring it to a boil. Add the broccoli, cover the pan, and boil for only 2 minutes. Drain.

Bring a large pan of salted water to a boil. When it boils, add the spaghetti.

Meanwhile, heat the olive oil in a large frying pan, add the garlic, and cook over a low heat for a minute or two, until just browned. Add the broccoli and stir it around for a minute, over the heat. Sprinkle with sea salt and plenty of black pepper and turn off the heat.

The spaghetti should be ready in 7–10 minutes, less if it's fresh. It should be cooked through but still with a slight bite to it (al dente). Drain it, rinse it through with running hot water, and put it in a warmed serving bowl. Mix in the broccoli and garlic and serve immediately.

Have the sea salt and black pepper grinders on the table to season the spaghetti if necessary, and, if you like, a bowl of freshly grated Parmesan cheese to sprinkle over it.

## Pasta with Pesto Sauce

*Serves 4*

> 350 g./12 oz. thin flat pasta
> 2 tablespoons crème fraîche (or heavy cream)
> 25 g./1 oz. butter
> salt and pepper
>
> SAUCE
> 3–4 garlic cloves, peeled
> 1 large bunch fresh basil, cleaned and dried
> 4–5 tablespoons freshly grated Parmesan cheese
> 3–4 tablespoons good olive oil

First make the pesto sauce. Pound the garlic in a mortar until smooth, and then add the basil leaves and crush them into the garlic until they form a paste. Beat in the cheese with a fork and begin to add the olive oil, drop by drop.

Cook the pasta in plenty of boiling salted water, until just firm (al dente). Drain well and toss in a warmed bowl with the cream and butter and plenty of salt and pepper.

Stir in the pesto sauce and serve immediately.

## Tagliatelle with Cheese and Garlic

*Serves 4*

    350 g./12 oz. tagliatelle
    2 tablespoons olive oil
    75 g./3 oz. each of bel paese, mozzarella, and dolcelatte, all diced
    75 g./3 oz. Parmesan, grated
    2 cloves garlic, crushed
    1 small bunch basil, chopped
    salt and black pepper

Boil the tagliatelle for 8 minutes or until al dente. Drain.

Heat the oil in a heavy-based pan and toss the pasta in it. Add the cheeses and mix well over a gentle heat. Mix in the garlic and basil, and season to taste with salt and lots of black pepper. Carry on tossing for a minute or two to allow all the tastes to blend, and then serve on warm plates.

# FISH, MEAT, AND POULTRY

## Cod Stew

*Serves 4*

- 450–750 g./1–1½ lb. cod fillet, skinned and cut into 4 pieces
- salt and pepper
- 1 clove garlic, crushed
- 2 tablespoons olive oil
- 2 onions, sliced
- 450 g./1 lb. beefsteak tomatoes, skinned and chopped
- 2 teaspoons chopped fresh thyme
- 2 teaspoons soy sauce

Sprinkle the cod with salt and pepper and rub all over with the garlic. Set aside for 15 minutes.

Meanwhile, heat the oil in a large saucepan, add the onions, and fry gently until soft.

Add the tomatoes, thyme, and soy sauce and bring to a boil. Then partly cover and simmer for 10 minutes, until pulpy.

Add the fish, and then cover and cook for 12–15 minutes, until tender.

Serve with steamed or boiled potatoes or yams.

## Moules Marinière

*Serves 4*

> 1.5 kg./3 lb. large mussels
> 300 ml./½ pint dry white wine
> 1 tablespoon white wine vinegar
> 3 shallots, finely chopped
> 1 large garlic clove, crushed
> pepper
> 1 bouquet garni
> pat of butter
> 3 basil leaves, shredded

Scrape and clean the mussels.

In a large pot, combine all the ingredients except the mussels and basil. Bring to a boil and simmer for 4 minutes.

Add the mussels to the stock, cover, and cook quickly until all the mussels are opened, stirring once or twice. Discard any mussel that has not opened (it's spoiled).

Add the shredded basil, check the seasoning, and serve at once.

# Prawns with Spicy Egg Rice

*Serves 4*

> 3 tablespoons oil
> 1 onion, chopped
> 1 clove garlic, crushed
> 1 teaspoon ground coriander
> ½ teaspoon chili powder
> 1 teaspoon ground cumin
> 1 teaspoon curry powder
> 250 g./8 oz. peeled prawns
> 1 tablespoon soy sauce
> 125 g./4 oz. frozen peas
> 250 g./8 oz. long-grain rice, cooked
> salt and pepper
>
> OMELETTE
> 1 free-range egg, beaten
> 1 tablespoon chopped spring onion to garnish
> salt and pepper

Heat 2 tablespoons of oil in a large pan, add the onion, and fry until softened.

Add the garlic, coriander, chili powder, cumin, and curry powder, stir well, and cook for 1 minute.

Stir in the prawns until they're well coated, and then add the soy sauce, peas, 4 tablespoons of water, and the salt and pepper. Cook for 2 minutes.

Add the rice, mix in well, and then cover and cook gently until thoroughly heated through.

Meanwhile, make the omelette. Beat together the egg, 2 tablespoons of water, and some of the salt and pepper. Heat the remaining oil in a frying pan, add the egg, and cook until just set. Slide on to a plate, roll up, and cut into strips.

Turn the rice mixture onto a warmed serving dish and arrange the egg strips on top. Sprinkle with the spring onion and serve immediately.

## Stuffed Sardines

*Serves 4*

> 24 small fresh sardines, scaled
> flour
> salt and pepper
> 1 kg./2 lb. fresh spinach
> olive oil
> 1 medium onion
> 3 cloves garlic, finely chopped
> ½ teaspoon grated nutmeg
> 1 tablespoon thyme, finely chopped
> 75 g./3 oz. white breadcrumbs, soaked in milk
> 2 tablespoons chervil, chopped
> 2 tablespoons chives, chopped
> 2 free-range eggs, beaten

Preheat the oven to 450°F.

Cut the heads off the fish, slit them along the belly, and remove the guts and backbones, leaving the tails attached. Open and flatten the fish. Sprinkle the skin side with a little flour and salt and pepper.

Wash the spinach thoroughly and cook in a covered saucepan until tender. Drain. Squeeze out the excess moisture and chop the spinach finely.

Cook the onion and garlic in oil until soft. Add the spinach, nutmeg, and thyme and continue cooking for 5 minutes.

Let the onion and spinach mixture cool, and then stir in the squeezed-out breadcrumbs, chervil, chives, and eggs. Scoop heaped spoonfuls onto the interior (flesh) side of 12 sardines and press the other 12 on top. The tails of the two layers of fish should be pointing in opposite directions.

Place the sardines in a well-oiled baking dish, brush with oil, and bake for 10 minutes, or until brown and tender.

## Trout with Garlic and Herb Sauce

*Serves 4*

    2 tablespoons olive oil
    4 ripe tomatoes, skinned and chopped
    3 anchovy fillets, finely chopped (optional)
    4 trout, each weighing about 250 g./8 oz., gutted
    2 tablespoons pesto sauce (see page 119)
    salt and pepper
    parsley sprigs to garnish

Heat the oil in a frying pan, add the tomatoes, and fry gently for about 5 minutes. Season with pepper and add the anchovies, if using. Keep warm.

Season the trout inside and out with salt and pepper. Cook under a preheated medium broiler for 5–6 minutes on each side.

Just before serving, stir the pesto into the tomato sauce. Pour a little sauce over each fish and garnish with parsley sprigs.

# Chicken with Ginger and Garlic Yogurt

*Serves 4*

1.75 kg./3½ lb. roasting chicken (free range)
150 g./5 oz. (½ of a small container) of natural yogurt
juice of half a lemon
2 tablespoons tomato purée
50 g./2 oz. root ginger
1 clove garlic, crushed

Preheat the oven to 400°F.

Joint the chicken and lay the joints, skin-side up, in an ovenproof dish.

Mix together the yogurt, lemon juice, and tomato purée.

Peel the ginger and grate it directly into the yogurt mixture.

Mix in the garlic and spoon the mixture over the chicken pieces.

Put the chicken in the oven and cook for 45 minutes, or until the skin crisps and browns.

Serve straight from the dish, with basmati rice.

## Chicken Baked in a Salty Garlic Crust with Pink Sauce

A rich dish, for special occasions. The combination of tomatoes and cream gives the sauce its glorious pink color.

*Serves 4–5*

> 1.25–1.5 kg./2½–3 lb. fresh free-range chicken
> 6 cloves garlic, peeled and roughly chopped
> coarse salt
>
> SAUCE
> 700 g./1½ lb. tomatoes
> 50 g./2 oz. butter
> 2.5 cm./1 inch piece fresh ginger, peeled and finely chopped
> 150 ml./¼ pint heavy cream
> salt
> cayenne pepper

Preheat the oven to 450°F.

Choose a deep, ovenproof casserole with a tight-fitting lid, in which the chicken will fit with 1–2 inches to spare all around. Line the base of the dish with two layers of foil, bringing it up well over the edges.

Put the chopped garlic in the body cavity of the chicken. Sprinkle a thickish layer of coarse salt into the dish, put the chicken in breast-side downward, and then pour in enough salt to bury the bird completely.

Cover the dish and place in the center of the oven for about 2 hours, or until cooked.

Shortly before the chicken is cooked, make the sauce. Put the tomatoes in a bowl, pour boiling water over them, leave for a minute, and then drain and peel the tomatoes and chop them up very small.

Melt the butter in a heavy saucepan over medium heat. Add the chopped ginger and the tomatoes and let them bubble gently in the open saucepan for 10–15 minutes, until they are cooked and mushy. Put to the side for later use.

When the chicken is ready, take the casserole dish out of the oven and spoon the top layer of salt into a large bowl. Then lift out the chicken with the help of the foil, tipping all the rest of the salt into the bowl as you do so. Wipe any remaining grains of salt off the chicken and put it on a serving dish in a low oven to keep warm while you finish the sauce.

Using a wooden spoon, carefully rub the tomato and ginger mixture through a sieve into another saucepan. Stir in the cream and boil, continuing to stir for 3–4 minutes, until the sauce thickens slightly. Remove from the heat and season to taste with salt and cayenne pepper.

Just before serving, pour the sauce evenly over the chicken.

## Madhur Jaffrey's Chicken in Garlic and Onion Sauce

*Serves 4–6*

- 1.25 kg./2½ lb. chicken joints
- 350 g./12 oz. onions, peeled
- 4 cm./1½ inch cube fresh ginger, peeled and coarsely chopped
- 6 cloves garlic, peeled
- 7 tablespoons vegetable oil
- 1 tablespoon ground coriander seeds
- 1 tablespoon ground cumin seeds
- ½ teaspoon ground turmeric
- ¼–½ teaspoon cayenne pepper
- 4 tablespoons plain yogurt
- 225 g./8 oz. tomatoes, peeled and very finely chopped
- 2 teaspoons salt
- ½ teaspoon garam masala
- 1 tablespoon fresh cilantro, finely chopped, to garnish

Skin the chicken and cut into serving pieces.

Chop half the onions coarsely. Cut the remaining onions into halves, lengthwise, and then crosswise into very thin slices. Put the chopped onions, ginger, and garlic into a blender or food processor. Blend until you have a paste.

Heat the oil in a large wide pot or frying pan over a medium heat. When hot, put in the sliced onions. Stir and fry until they're a deep reddish brown. Remove the onions with a slotted spoon, squeezing them out to leave behind as much of the oil as possible. Put the onions onto a plate and set aside.

Take the pot off the heat. Put in the blended paste and return to the heat. Stir and fry the paste until brown; it will take about 3–4 minutes.

Add the coriander seeds, cumin, turmeric, and cayenne pepper, stirring once.

Stir in 1 tablespoon of the yogurt for about 30 seconds, or until it's has been incorporated into the sauce. Continue to add the rest of the yogurt in the same way, a tablespoon at a time.

Put in the chicken pieces and stir them around for 1 minute.

Pour in 1 pint of water, and then add the tomatoes and salt. Stir to mix and bring to a simmer. Cover, turn the heat to low, and cook for 20 minutes.

Add the garam masala and the fried onions. Mix well. Cook, uncovered, over a medium heat for 7–8 minutes, or until the sauce reduces and thickens.

Skim off the fat and place the chicken in a warm serving dish. Sprinkle the fresh cilantro over the top before serving.

## Poussins Stuffed with Garlic and Olives

*Serves 4*

2 small chickens weighing 700 g /1½ lb. each, or 5 poussins/rock Cornish game hens weighing 350–400 g./12–14 oz. each
75 g./3 oz. unsmoked bacon, finely chopped
salt and pepper
2 heads garlic, unpeeled

STUFFING
the chicken giblets (heart, gizzard, and liver), chopped
2 cloves garlic, finely chopped
2 slices bread, soaked in milk and squeezed out
150 g./6 oz. black olives, pitted and crushed

Preheat the oven to 375°F.

Mix all the stuffing ingredients thoroughly and stuff the birds. Sew up the cavities and truss well.

Saute the chopped bacon until the fat runs. Set aside the fried bacon, brush the birds with the fat, season with salt and pepper, and place birds breast-side up in an oiled casserole (preferably earthenware) just large enough to hold them. Push the garlic between the birds and cook for about 30–40 minutes, or until the juice from the thigh runs clear.

When the birds are cooked, either scoop out the stuffing and serve separately or cut the birds in half with poultry shears and leave the stuffing inside.

Test the garlic heads with the point of a knife. If not completely tender, place in boiling water for 5–7 minutes.

When soft, squeeze the garlic into the pan juices, stir well, and spoon over the birds.

Serve hot, garnished with the fried bacon pieces if desired.

## Lamb with Garlic Tarts

A special dish for dinner parties

**Serves 6**

- 1 leg of lamb
- 2 cloves garlic, sliced in strips
- 5 or 6 anchovies, cut in pieces
- olive oil
- salt and freshly ground black pepper
- 10 garlic heads
- 3 tablespoons light cream
- 1 tablespoon tomato purée
- 6 small prebaked pastry shells

Preheat the oven to 450°F.

Make small deep stabs with a pointed knife all over the lamb and press into them the slices of garlic and anchovy pieces. Brush the lamb with olive oil and rub a very little salt and lots of ground pepper into the skin.

Place the roast on a rack over the vegetables, so that the juices can drip through. Wrap the whole garlic heads in foil and place beside the roast. Roast for the first 10 minutes in a very hot oven, and then turn the heat down to 375°F and continue roasting for 15–20 minutes per pound, or until cooked to taste.

Allow the lamb to rest in a warm place for 20 minutes before carving.

Meanwhile, make the sauce. Test the garlic heads with the point of a knife. If not completely tender, place in boiling water for 5–7 minutes. When soft, cut the root ends off the garlic cloves and squeeze the paste into a bowl. Beat until creamy with 5–6 tablespoons of the juices from the roasting pan, the thin cream, and the tomato purée. (If you have had to boil the garlic, some of its cooking liquid could be used to thin the sauce if necessary.) Add plenty of pepper (and salt, if needed).

Spoon some of the sauce into the prebaked pastry shells and serve hot around the roast.

# Further Reading

Ayanoglu, Byron. *The New Vegetarian Gourmet*. Robert Rose, Inc., 1996.

Buchman, Dian Dincin, with the Herb Society. *Herbal Medicine —The Natural Way to Stay Well*. Rider, 1996.

David, Elizabeth. *Summer Cooking*. Penguin, 1987.

Forbes, Leslie. *Taste of Provence*. Chronicle Books, 1991.

Jaffrey, Madhur. *Madhur Jaffrey's Indian Cookery*. BBC Books, 1982.

Saynor, Reg. *The Garlic Effect*. Hodder & Stoughton, 1995.

Smith, Delia. *Delia Smith's Complete Cookery Course*. BBC Books, 1992.

Wilen, Joan, and Lydia Wilen, *Garlic—Nature's Super Healer*. Prentice Hall, 1997.

# Index

Acne, 30–31
AIDS, 21
Ajoene, 24
Alcohol, and health, 63–64
Allergies, 39–41
Allicin, 3, 8, 24, 70–71
Allinase, 3
Anemia, 31
Anger, 64, 65–66
Angina pectoris, 10, 18–21
Animal bites, 31
Antioxidant activity, 11
Arteriosclerosis, 10, 11–12, 52
Arthritis, 31
Aspirin, 18
Asthma, 32
Athlete's foot, 32–33, 46–47

Baird, Ian, 15–16

Barlow, Philip, 71
Beeton, Mrs., 2
Bites
  animal, 31
  insect, 43
Blisters, 33
Blood circulation, 24–28
Blood pressure, 21–23
Boils, 33
Bronchitis, 33
Buchman, Dian Dincin, 29–30, 32
Burns, 34

Calf pain, 25, 26
Cancer, 23–24
  and dietary fiber, 58
Candidiasis (thrush), 34–35
Cheese recipes, 102–103
Chicken recipes, 129–35
Chilblains, 35

Chinese garlic, 71
Cholesterol, 10–11, 12, 13, 52, 53–55
Clayton, Caroline, 35
Cold sores, 36
Colds, 35–36
Constipation, 36
Contraceptive pills, and thrombosis, 26, 27
Coronary heart disease. *See* Heart disease
Culpeper, Nicholas, 2
Cystitis, 36–37

Deep vein thrombosis, 25–28
Dehydration, 66–68
Diabetes, 28
Diallyl disulfide, 23
Diarrhea, 37–38
Diet
　and health, 51–60
　ideal, 59–60
Digestive problems, 38
Dip and sauce recipes, 105–12

Earache, 38
Ernst, Edzard, 12, 13, 71
Estrogen, 25–27
Exercise, and health, 60–62

Fatigue, 39
Fats (lipids) in blood, 10–11, 53–55

Fiber in diet, 56–59
Fish recipes, 122–28
Flu, 35–36
Food preparation methods, 60

Garlic
　and common ailments, 6–7, 29–49
　composition, 3
　and health, 4–5, 9–28
　health benefits, 4–5, 9–28, 29–49
　history, 1–3
　preparations, 49–50
　recipes, 76–137
　supplements, 70–73
　use, 70–73
Garlic breath, 73
Garlic Information Center, 3, 4–5, 6–7
Garlic oil, 70
Garlic poultice, 50
Garlic tea, 50
Garlic water, 50
Gum problems, 39

Hangovers, 39
Hannaford, Philip, 26–27, 28
Hay fever, 39–41
HDL (high density lipoprotein), 11
Headache, 41
Health benefits, of garlic, 4–5, 9–28, 29–49

Heart disease, 9–21, 51–53
  and dietary fiber, 58–59
Hemorrhoids, 41
Herpes, 41
High blood pressure, 21–23
High fiber diet, 56–59
Hippocrates, 36
History, of garlic, 1–3
HIV, 21
HRT (hormone replacement therapy), 25–27

Immune system, 21, 23
Impotence, 41–43
Insect bites and stings, 43
Insulin, 58

Jock itch, 46–47

Kwai garlic tablets, 71

Lalitha Thomas' enhanced garlic formula, 49
LDL (low density lipoprotein), 11
Lipids (fats) in blood, 10–11, 53–55

Mastitis, 43–44
Meat recipes, 136–37
Mediterranean diet, 59–60
Messegue, Maurice, 42–43
Minerals, in garlic, 3
Moniliasis, 34–35
Monounsaturated fats, 53, 55

Morning sickness, 45

Neil, Andrew, 22

Odor, and garlic, 3, 73
Onions, 71

Pasta recipes, 116–20
Petrie, Sir William, 2
Piotrowski, F. G., 23
Pliny, 2
PMS, 45–46
Polyunsaturated fats, 53–54, 55
Preparations, garlic, 49–50

Recipes, 76–137
Relaxing, and health, 64–66
Ringworm, 46–47
Russians, and garlic, 2

S-Allylcysteine, 23
Salad recipes, 84–89
Salt in diet, 23, 55–56
Saturated fats, 53–55
Sauce and dip recipes, 105–12
Saynor, Reg, 36, 71
Sciatica, 48
Silagy, Christopher, 22
Sinusitis, 48
Smoking, and health, 62–63
Sore throat, 48
Soup recipes, 78–83

Sugar in diet, 55–56
Sulfides, 8
Sunburn, 48–49
Supplements, garlic, 70–73

Thomas' enhanced garlic
 formula, 49
Thrombosis, 25–28
Thrush, 34–35
Tinea (ringworm),
 46–47
Tinea corporis, 46–47
Tinea cruris, 46–47

Tinea pedis, 32–33, 46–47
Toothache, 49
Type A/B behavior, 64–65

Vaginal candidiasis, 34–35
Vegetable recipes, 92–99
Vitamins, in garlic, 3

Water, and health, 66–68
Watercress, 23
Wilen, Joan and Lydia, 38,
 73
Wren, Barbara, 66, 67–68

## About the Author

Karen Evennett has been a freelance journalist for over ten years and specializes in writing about health and relationships for women's magazines. *Garlic: The Natural Remedy* is Karen's fifth book. She is the author of *The PMS Diet Book*, *Coping Successfully with PMS*, *Coping Successfully with Your Cervical Smear*, and *Women's Health: An Essential Guide for the Modern Woman*. Karen loves good food, and her husband, Steve, a chef, has worked in some of London's top restaurants. They have two daughters, Coco and Bella, and live in Surrey, England.

# Ulysses Press Health Books

## A Natural Approach Books

Written in a friendly, nontechnical style, *A Natural Approach* books address specific health issues and show you how to take an active part in your own treatment. Whether you suffer from panic attacks, endometriosis or depression, each book will provide you with a thorough understanding of your condition and detail organic solutions that offer immediate relief for your symptoms and effectively remedy their underlying causes.

Believing that disease is more than a combination of symptoms, these books offer integrated mind/body programs that take a positive, preventative approach. Since traditional drug therapy is not always the best solution (and can sometimes be the problem), these guides show how to use alternative treatments to supplement or replace conventional medicine.

ANXIETY & DEPRESSION
ISBN 1-56975-118-8, 144 pp, $9.95

ENDOMETRIOSIS
ISBN 1-56975-088-2, 184 pp, $9.95

FREE YOURSELF FROM
TRANQUILIZERS
& SLEEPING PILLS
ISBN 1-56975-074-2, 192 pp, $9.95

IRRITABLE BLADDER &
INCONTINENCE
ISBN 1-56975-089-0, 108 pp, $8.95

IRRITABLE BOWEL SYNDROME
ISBN 1-56975-030-0, 240 pp, $12.95

MIGRAINES
ISBN 1-56975-140-4, 156 pp, $8.95

PANIC ATTACKS
ISBN 1-56975-045-9, 148 pp, $9.95

## The Natural Remedy Books

As home remedies and alternative treatments become increasingly accepted into the medical mainstream, people want information—not just hype and unproven claims—about the remedies they see in health food stores. *The Natural Remedy* books detail how these natural remedies have been used throughout history and how to safely incorporate them into an overall plan for maintaining good health.

CIDER VINEGAR
ISBN 1-56975-141-2, 120 pp, $8.95

GARLIC
ISBN 1-56975-097-1, 120 pp, $9.95

# Discover Handbooks

Easy to follow and authoritative, *Discover Handbooks* reveal an array of alternative therapies from around the world and demonstrate how to incorporate them into a program of good health.

Each book opens with information on the history and principles of the particular technique, then presents practical and straightforward guidance on ways in which it can be applied. Offering the tools needed to achieve and maintain an optimal state of health, the approach is one of personal improvement and self-reliance. Each of the books features: an introduction to the discipline; an explanation of its philosophy; step-by-step guide to its implementation; clear diagrams and charts; and case studies.

DISCOVER AYURVEDA
ISBN 1-56975-081-5, 128 pp, $8.95

DISCOVER COLOR THERAPY
ISBN 1-56975-093-9, 144 pp, $8.95

DISCOVER ESSENTIAL OILS
ISBN 1-56975-080-7, 128 pp, $8.95

DISCOVER FLOWER ESSENCES
ISBN 1-56975-099-8, 120 pp, $8.95

DISCOVER MEDITATION
ISBN 1-56975-113-7, 144 pp, $8.95

DISCOVER NUTRITIONAL THERAPY
ISBN 1-56975-135-8, 120 pp, $8.95

DISCOVER OSTEOPATHY
ISBN 1-56975-115-3, 132 pp, $8.95

DISCOVER REFLEXOLOGY
ISBN 1-56975-112-9, 132 pp, $8.95

DISCOVER SHIATSU
ISBN 1-56975-082-3, 128 pp, $8.95

# The Ancient and Healing Arts Books

*The Ancient and Healing Arts* books recount the development of healing art forms that have been used for thousands of years. Beautifully illustrated with full color on every page, they discuss the benefits of these time-honored techniques and offer detailed instructions on their use.

THE ANCIENT AND HEALING ART OF AROMATHERAPY
ISBN 1-56975-094-7, 96 pp, $14.95

THE ANCIENT AND HEALING ART OF CHINESE HERBALISM
ISBN 1-56975-139-0, 96 pp, $14.95

# Other Health Titles

THE BOOK OF KOMBUCHA
ISBN 1-56975-049-1, 160 pp, $11.95
Explains the benefits of and addresses concerns about Kombucha, the widely used Chinese "tea mushroom."

HEALING REIKI: REUNITE MIND, BODY AND SPIRIT
WITH HEALING ENERGIES
ISBN 1-56975-162-5, 124 pp, $16.95
Examines the meaning, perception and history of this ancient healing technique while providing practical tips for giving and receiving Reiki.

HEPATITIS C: A PERSONAL GUIDE TO GOOD HEALTH
ISBN 1-56975-091-2, 172 pp, $12.95
Identifies the causes and symptoms of hepatitis C and presents conventional and alternative treatments for coping with the disease.

KNOW YOUR BODY: THE ATLAS OF ANATOMY
ISBN 1-56975-021-1, 160 pp, $12.95
Presents a full-color guide to the structure of the human body.

MOOD FOODS
ISBN 1-56975-023-8, 192 pp, $11.95
Shows how the foods you eat influence your emotions and behavior.

YOUR NATURAL PREGNANCY: A GUIDE TO COMPLEMENTARY THERAPIES
ISBN 1-56975-059-9, 240 pp, $16.95
Details alternative therapies ranging from aromatherapy to yoga that can benefit pregnant women.

---

*To order these books call 800-377-2542, fax 510-601-8307 or write to Ulysses Press, P.O. Box 3440, Berkeley, CA 94703-3440. All retail orders are shipped free of charge. California residents must include sales tax. Allow two to three weeks for delivery.*